Le Personal Coach

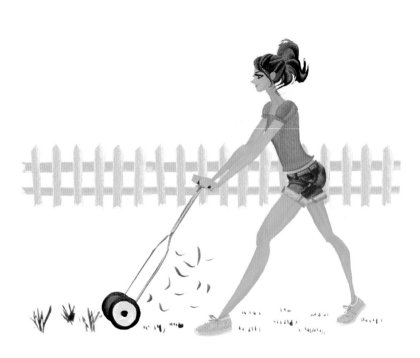

Le Personal Coach

A French Trainer's Simple Secrets for Getting Fit and Slim without the Gym

Valérie Orsoni

Celebrity Coach and Founder of LeBootCamp®

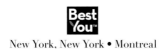

New York, New York • Montreal

Project Editor Ellen Michaud
Copy Editor Barbara Booth
Interior Design Vertigo Design NYC
Cover Designer Jennifer Tokarski
Cover Photos Mikel Healey
Author Photo Mano
Illustrations Masaki Ryo
Senior Art Director George McKeon
Executive Editor, Trade Publishing Dolores York
Manufacturing Manager Elizabeth Dinda
Associate Publisher, Trade Publishing Rosanne McManus
President and Publisher, Trade Publishing Harold Clarke

Library of Congress Cataloging-in-Publication Data
Orsoni, Valérie.
Le personal coach : a French trainer's simple secrets for getting fit and slim without the gym / by Valérie Orsoni.
    p. cm.
  ISBN 978-1-60652-200-4
1. Physical fitness. 2. Physical fitness--Nutritional aspects. 3. Health. I. Title.
  RA781.O77 2011
  613.7--dc22
                                2010034397

We are committed to both the quality of our products and the service we provide to our customers. We value your comments, so please feel free to contact us.

    Best You Books
    The Reader's Digest Association, Inc.
    Adult Trade Publishing
    44 S. Broadway
    White Plains, NY 10601

Printed in China

1 3 5 7 9 10 8 6 4 2

NOTE TO OUR READERS
The information in this book should not be substituted for, or used to alter, medical therapy without your doctor's advice. For a specific health problem, consult your physician for guidance.

To my son, Baptiste, who brings out the sun
from behind the clouds for me.

. . . .

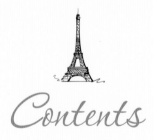

Contents

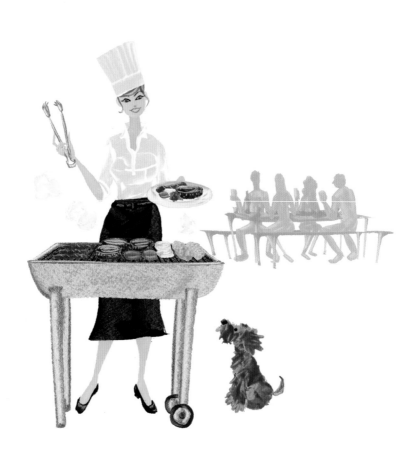

Foreword

Valérie Orsoni is my favorite personal coach. She has the freshest approach to fitness and weight loss seen in years.

As a caring mom who works full-time outside the home, she understands firsthand the constraints of work and family on women's lives, and she has developed a strategy for women to get fit and lose weight without adding one more minute to their busy days—no trips to the gym are required! And her strategies work. In fact, 92 percent of the women in Valérie's program have lost an average of 26 pounds—and never regained it!

Her secret? She's figured out how to integrate the most butt-tightening, breast-lifting, and ab-strengthening moves into everything from emptying the dishwasher to folding laundry, watching TV with the kids, hanging out at a kid's soccer practice, even while communicating with colleagues at work.

These moves, combined with proper nutrition and the commitment to a good night's sleep, will help women effortlessly reshape, rebuild, and renew their bodies.

—**Dr. Oz Garcia**
New York City

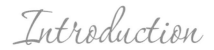

Introduction

Everyone—your doctor, your mother, the receptionist at your kids' school, even Oprah—tells you to exercise. But no one is telling you how you're supposed to work it into a day that's crammed with work, carpools, and laundry from 6:00 A.M. until midnight. But I can—by showing you how to integrate exercise, movement, and good food into every corner of your life. In fact, by using the hundreds of tricks, tips, and tasty recipes in this book, you can effortlessly reshape, rebuild, and renew your body in no time at all. What's more, you can achieve this without adding another minute to your busy day.

How? From doing toilet squats in the restroom to discreetly working your thighs at a traffic light, this book takes a fresh look at what burns calories and helps build a fabulous body. It may sound complicated, but it's really nothing more than child's play. My program takes little or no time away from jobs and family.

A key reason my program is so successful is my "25th hour" concept. It's what I originally created for my celebrity clients because they were always saying, "I don't have time to go to the gym. I'm always traveling. I have a crazy schedule." So I decided to create exercises that range from 1 to 15 minutes, like small routines that can be done anywhere—at work, in the car, on vacation—anytime.

So now I contract my glutes while sitting in the office, contract my abs while on the subway, work on my triceps in the bathtub, and walk rather than drive to meetings and appointments whenever I can. And if each of us routinely worked these drills into our daily habits, we would seamlessly integrate an extra hour's worth of exercise into our lives—just as though we had gained a 25th hour in the day. Then there would be no reason to feel guilty about not getting to the gym!

If actress Angelina Jolie can rely on integrative exercises such as these to keep her in shape while on the go, why can't you? It's a great way to optimize every moment to work your muscles and keep them toned. Practical and simple, these are habits that you soon won't be able to live without—and you will begin to notice visible results after just one month.

A second reason my program is so successful is that it's flexible: Like this piece of advice? Then follow it! Don't like that one? No problem; opt for an alternative!

In addition, I insist that my clients eat well. One of these days, I'm going to turn all my favorite recipes into a cookbook. But in the meantime, I've included "Bon Appétit!"—a selection of quick-and-easy recipes that help my body look good and stay fabulously healthy.

No way will I give up good food! I am an epicurean of the highest level. I would sell my soul for a glass of sauternes. When I go to Paris, I enjoy the macaroons from Fauchon. (My favorite? The violet macaroons.) But before enjoying these famous little delights, I eat 5 almonds to send a strong signal of fat/protein intake to my brain and—*voilà!*—I store less fat than my neighbor who opts for grabbing sweet stuff on an empty stomach.

Once you become aware of these easy but valuable tips, they will quickly become habit. Soon you can have the body you want, live your life without having to deprive yourself of good food, and most of all, enjoy some of life's greatest pleasures.

So no more excuses! Whether you're at work, at home, in your car, on vacation, or on a plane, there is no reason you can't reshape, rebuild, and renew your body.

Happy reading!

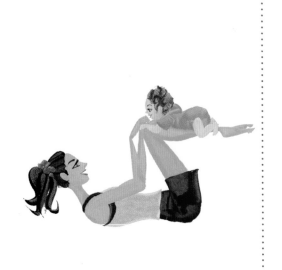
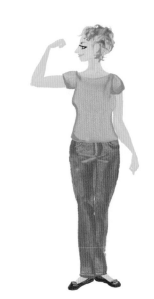
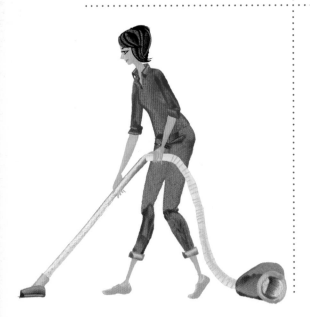
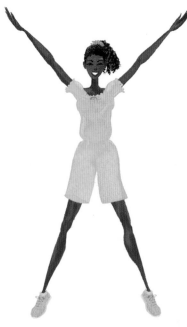

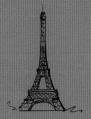

Les Secrets du Coach

Ever wonder why French women such as *Pirates of the Caribbean*'s Astrid Berges-Frisbey or *Chocolat*'s Juliette Binoche have such sexy derrières, lifted breasts, and supple arms? Like all French women, they know Les Secrets du Coach—quick strategies you can work into everything from talking on the phone and attending your kids' soccer games to emptying the dishwasher and eating almonds. Ready to hear what they are? Just turn the page!

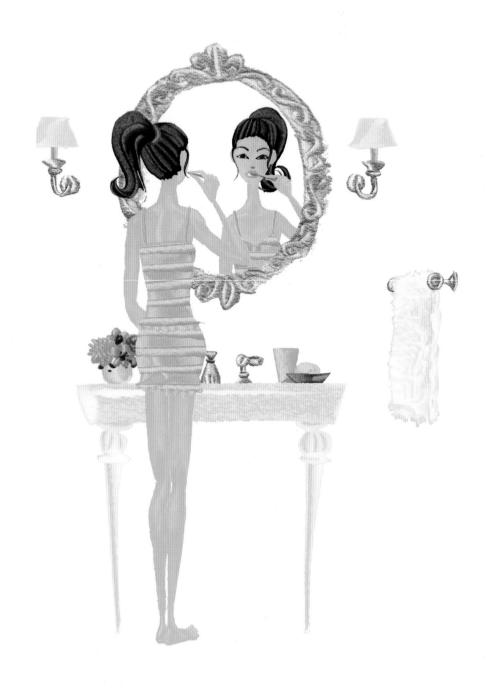

Catch the Brazilian curve!

Want to have a nice bottom to fill that summer swimsuit?

Stand up straight and bend your knees slightly. Keep your abs tight and your back straight (no arching) as you tilt your hips forward while contracting your glutes. Finish the move by pulling your hips back. Make sure you give an extra hard squeeze when you push your hips forward.

QUICK TRICK!

Do the Brazilian while brushing your teeth. Since you spend, on average, 6 minutes a day brushing your teeth, you have 6 extra minutes every day to work on your glutes. That's 42 minutes per week worth of butt squeezes, the equivalent of a booty class at the gym without the sweat. How easy can an exercise get?

Build killer thighs

Bring a small ball to your workplace. When sitting, put it between your legs at knee level. Squeeze and hold the squeeze. Do this 50 times a day—gradually increasing to 100 times a day. Your inner thighs will firm up beautifully. If you're sitting in a cubicle or in an open space where people can see you squeezing rapidly, then just hold the squeeze for 1 minute, or until it burns, and repeat throughout the day.

LE PETIT SECRET *Nutrition researchers have shown that eating an apple about 15 minutes before a meal will reduce your appetite.*

GRAB & GO! *Reach for juicy apples to satisfy the need for a snack—and get a healthy dose of disease prevention at the same time. Apples contain quercetin, a flavonoid antioxidant that protects cells against wear and tear that can contribute to chronic conditions such as heart disease and cancer. Just make sure you buy organic apples so you don't need to peel them.*

Use your kids' practice time

Do you drive your kids to karate, baseball, or dance practice?
Great! But don't sit through every practice. Your kids can thrive without having you watch them every minute. Instead, take your sneakers with you and go for a fast-paced hour-long walk. If your children have 2 or 3 practices per week, you'll end up getting 2 to 3 hours of good, healthy cardio exercise!

DO IT NOW! *While waiting for your kids to finish practice, why not invite other parents to take a walk? It's a good opportunity to talk about what's happening with everyone's kids, it'll encourage you to stay on track, and they'll thank you for making them fitter.*

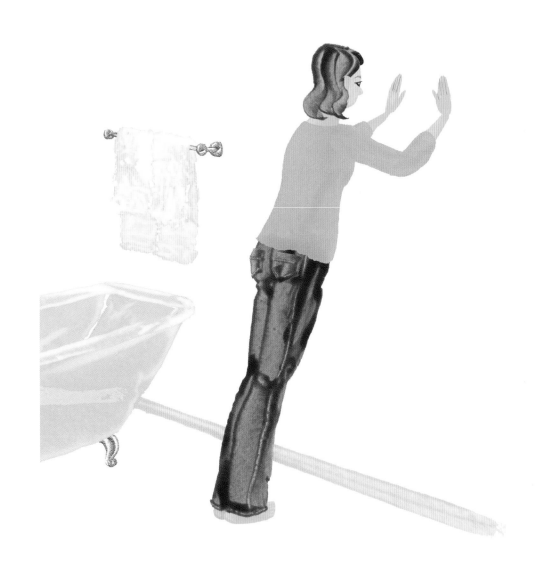

Push it!

Tone the backs of your arms with this easy move: Every time you go to the bathroom, stand in front of a wall with your arms straight at eye level. Place your palms on the wall and bend at the elbows to do 20 standing push-ups. Push your body back from the wall harder each time, moving slowly and maintaining control. Aim for 20 reps, and then repeat several times throughout the day.

QUICK TRICK!

For added benefit, rotate your hands inward so your fingers touch. To make it even more difficult, try to do one-arm push-ups, making sure your body is as flat and straight as a plank.

"French women do these exercises all day long. Now you know how they get such toned arms and lifted breasts!" —VALÉRIE

Fight fat with protein

Starting your meal with protein will help reduce the blood-sugar surge that usually occurs after eating refined carbs like white bread and potatoes. When your blood sugar increases that fast, your body is much more likely to store extra calories as fat at your next meal. It transforms your body into a fat-storing machine. Protein stacks the deck in your favor.

QUICK TRICK!

For a simple way to figure out portion size without weighing your food, picture a deck of cards on your plate. Then put your meal's protein—fish or meat, for example—in exactly that amount of space. That's all you need to build muscle. Anything more is extra calories that will go straight to your hips.

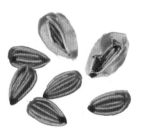

Get a natural breast lift!

You already know that breasts are not made of muscle and they can't be strengthened directly. But one of my very good friends who's a dancer at the famous Moulin Rouge in Paris shared this secret: Every morning after her shower, she does "chest presses" by pushing her hands together, palm against palm, 100 times. She starts by holding her arms at chest level; then she keeps moving them up until they're high above her head. This helps firm the supporting tissue around the breasts. It's like a natural breast lift and takes no more than 1 minute.

"When doing these presses, nothing prevents you from squeezing your glutes at the same time! I do both after applying my after-shower moisturizer, getting a breast lift at the same time the lotion is penetrating my skin!" —VALÉRIE

Keep your hands wet

There are some chores you'd be better off doing by hand.
And washing the dishes, which burns 78 calories per half hour, is
clearly one of them. Since it takes 3,500 calories burned to lose
1 pound of body fat, it's easy to see that you can lose 1 pound of
fat by washing your dishes by hand for 30 minutes a day over 45 days.

DO IT NOW! *One year's worth of washing the dishes by hand can knock 8 pounds off your body. Eight pounds!*

"I like to squeeze my glutes or dance in place when I do dishes as well. The soapsuds splash all over the place, but then I get to burn off even more calories by mopping the floor!" —VALÉRIE

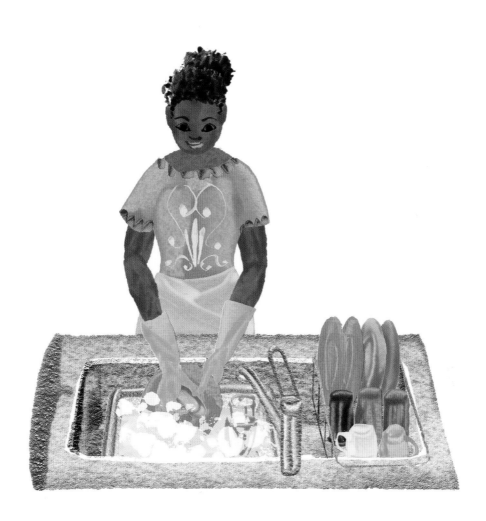

Walk while you talk

Do you have a cell phone? A cordless? How much time do you spend each day on one or the other? One hour? Two? More?

Can you imagine how many steps you could take each day if you were constantly walking while you talk? A lot!

So put a sticky note on your phone that says, "Walk while you talk." If you work from home, just walk around your home. If you're in an office, walk around or remain standing during the entire conversation as you shift your body weight from one leg to the other.

The point is to remain in motion. You'll burn more calories— and keep yourself more alert as well!

QUICK TRICK!

If you're in a place where you can't walk while on the phone, just tap your feet nonstop during the conversation. You'll burn 2 calories a minute. Think that's not much? Do the math. If you spend 2 hours a day on the phone, that's 120 calories you've burned. Keep it up and you'll lose a pound every month.

Party!

When you're invited to a party, what do you do? Do you remain seated for the entire evening? Do you stand by the buffet table talking?

Change your ways, girl! Stay away from that buffet table and dance! You'll have more fun, burn more calories, and get your cardio exercise all in one shot.

GRAB & GO! *Kill your appetite by grabbing a hard-boiled egg on your way out the door. Eat it on the way to your party.*

LE PETIT SECRET *Don't have time for a pedicure? Have dry feet that look bad in strappy party shoes? Try this trick the next time you go for a walk: Before you put on your socks, slather your feet with a moisturizing cream. Then put on your socks and shoes and hit the street. Combined with sweating, which opens your pores, the increased heat from walking will help the cream penetrate much better than if you had simply put it on before going to bed.*

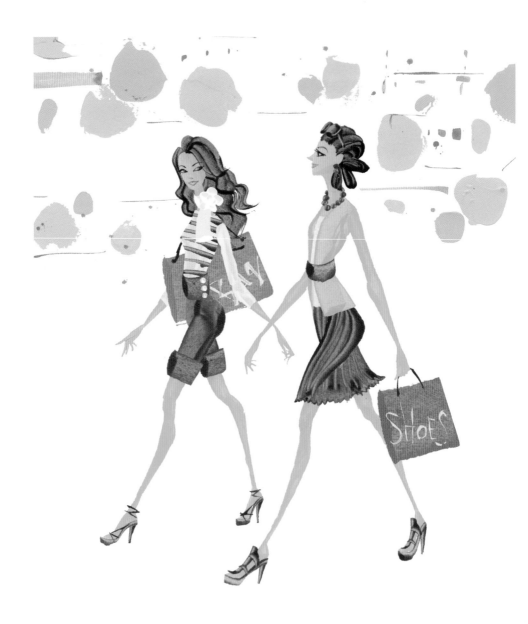

Shop and drop (pounds!)

Go to the mall at lunchtime and walk nonstop at a good pace.
Take your friends with you—and wear a pedometer! Walk for
1,000 steps the first day, then gradually work yourselves up to
5,000 steps over the lunch break. And don't stop to look at all
the tempting clothes—just walk!

DO IT NOW! *When you do go shopping, buy a blouse or pair of pants one size smaller than you actually wear. Toss this new piece of clothing in a spot where you'll see it constantly: on the back of the door in the bathroom, on the back of a chair in the kitchen. The fact that your brain will register this too-small piece of clothing every time you pass it will positively brainwash you into making the right food decisions—like not taking a second helping of that yummy dessert in the fridge!*

Ditch the "meal replacement" bars

Sold as "meal replacements" at the supermarket, the majority of these bars are loaded with saturated fat, genetically modified ingredients, and too many preservatives and artificial flavorings and colors to count. They're a great way to gain weight! Also, the fact that the brain is registering that we are eating something supposedly healthy and weight-loss friendly puts us in a position where we feel we can have a little bit more—which usually means we end up eating twice as much. The same applies to replacement drinks; we tend to add some additional foods to compensate for the lack of taste and "chewing."

GRAB & GO! *For those all-too-frequent moments when there's no time for dinner, keep a supply of turkey jerky in your handbag, car, desk—anywhere it's handy. A standard large pouch of jerky has 4 servings and will contain less than 3 percent total fat—with no saturated fat!—and a good amount of protein. Not only will it satisfy hunger, the time it takes to actually chew jerky will also give you enough time to feel full so you don't start craving a doughnut!*

ST☆R Rx

DEMI MOORE'S FLAT TUMMY

Demi defies the years with an amazing grace and a ripped body. If you want your abs to look like hers, work these easy moves into your life:

- Each time you pass through a door, suck in your upper and lower abs as hard as you can.

- While you're watching TV, at each commercial break do the V-Pilates: Without arching your back, sit on your bottom and raise both legs into the air, toes pointed, so your body forms the letter V. Hold for 30 seconds minimum; ideally for 1 minute.

- Before taking your shower every morning, do 100 crunches on your bedroom carpet or mat.

By making sure your abs are engaged throughout the day, you will develop a nice, flat tummy in no time.

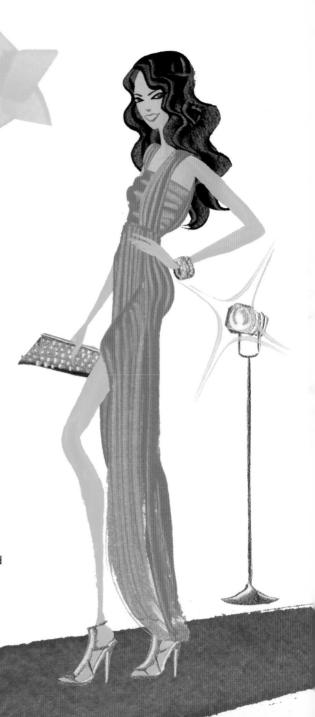

Eat good fat

All fat is not created equal. The fat in fish helps prevent heart disease. The fat in meat causes it. Plus, as a general rule, fish is leaner than meat to begin with. Try eating fish at least twice a week. (See my recipe for Wild Salmon en Papillote on page 156.)

QUICK TRICK!

Grill a little extra fish and stick it in the refrigerator for fish tacos or fish burgers the next night. Salsa is a great way to spice up a meal without introducing lots of extra calories.

GRAB & GO! *Smoked salmon rolls with a dollop of low-fat cream cheese are high-antioxidant/great protein/good-fat treats. Use them as an appetizer with friends, but hold back a few in the fridge for a day or so to eat as healthy snacks! (See my recipe on page 153.)*

"Shop for fresh fish or fish marked FAS—frozen at sea. Avoid overfished species, such as sturgeon, cod, halibut, and the mercury-loaded species—like tuna and shark." —VALÉRIE

The 21-day sugar cure

Refined sugar plays havoc with your blood sugar. And that can affect both your appetite and how your body stores food. To keep sugar cravings in check, don't go cold turkey. Instead, reduce the amount of sugar in beverages and foods a little every day. After about 21 days, your urge to eat and drink sugary foods and beverages should vanish. And you can cross refined sugar off your grocery list forever!

GRAB & GO! *Bananas contain 3 natural sugars—sucrose, fructose, and glucose. Combined with fiber, bananas give an instant sustained and substantial boost of energy (not to mention the much-needed potassium, which we use up when exercising). Just 2 bananas will provide enough energy for a strenuous 90-minute workout! (See my recipe for Banana Chips on page 145.)*

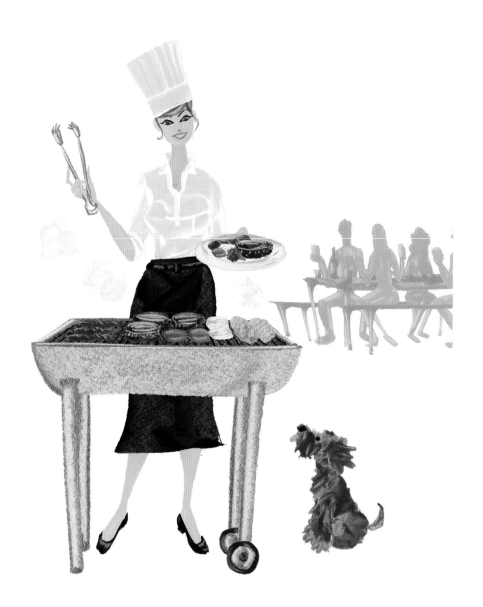

Be the rotisserie chef!

Taking care of the backyard barbecue will keep you far away from the temptingly rich goodies and high-calorie alcoholic beverages laid out on the picnic tables.

QUICK TRICK!
Try to make every minute count. While you're grilling steaks at your next barbecue, remember to suck in your stomach and squeeze those glutes!

DO IT NOW! *You'll burn 130 calories per hour vs. the 60 calories you'd burn if you were just sitting with friends.*

"When setting up for a barbecue, I make as many trips back and forth as possible, one for the meat, another for condiments... the trip for charcoal is the best. Hauling that heavy bag outside works my biceps and burns calories!" —VALÉRIE

Head for the bathroom every hour

That's right. Every hour. But before going to the bathroom itself, go for a walk around the block or around your building. This is little enough time not to interfere with your workday but long enough so that—if you do it every hour or so—you will have accumulated 60 minutes of walking a day without breaking a sweat!

DO IT NOW! *Having trouble remembering to walk? Get a dog. Or borrow your neighbors'. People who have a dog have been proven to weigh less than their dogless counterpart—mainly because they need to walk the dog a minimum of twice a day for 30 minutes each time. That burns about 300 calories right there! After 1 month and with a balanced diet, that's 3 pounds of fat lost. And if you lack motivation, your dog will make sure you don't forget!*

Sneak in a lunchtime walk

Having lunch with your coworkers? Choose to walk the 10 to 15 minutes to the restaurant. This will help you fit in about 30 minutes of daily walking time. Walking your way back to your workplace will also help with digestion and clear your mind before you start working again.

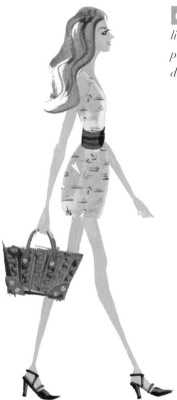

GRAB & GO! *Bring workplace snacks like mozzarella sticks, wrapped in an individual package, from home. You'll be less likely to devour enough to sabotage your diet.*

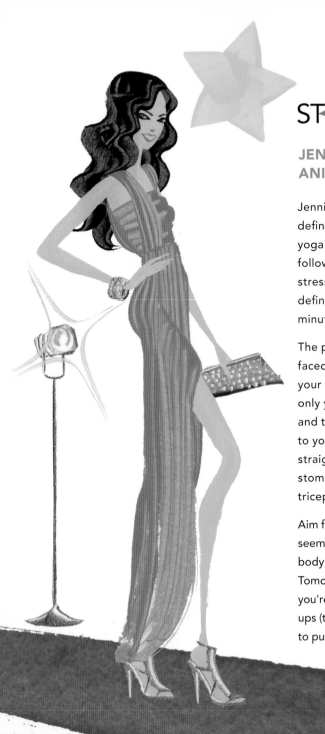

ST★R Rx

JENNIFER ANISTON'S ARMS

Jennifer Aniston owes her nicely defined triceps to an arduous yoga routine she religiously follows, no matter her level of stress. You, too, can get the same definition without sweating 90 minutes a day doing headstands.

The plank is your ally here. Lie facedown on a yoga mat and lift your body up, supporting it with only your elbows, forearms, hands, and toes. Keep your elbows close to your torso and keep your back straight as a plank. Zip up your stomach as well, and visualize your triceps supporting your entire body.

Aim for 1 minute, 3 times a day. If this seems too hard at first, go until your body starts shaking and count to 5. Tomorrow, add a few more seconds. If you're in good shape, add 5 easy push-ups (the ones you do on your knees, to put less pressure on your wrists).

Curb your thighs

Waiting at a red light to cross? Go up and down on and off the curb. Keep your feet flat so you mainly work your thighs. And keep an eye out for oncoming traffic!

QUICK TRICK!

If you're carrying a couple of shopping bags, ramp up the benefits of curb exercises by adding bicep curls. Just turn your palms up, slide a shopping bag handle over each one, then alternate lifting one bag and then the other. And of course, ignore the stares from the people waiting at the red light with you.

DO IT NOW! *Having trouble getting started? Just imagine the jealous eyes of friends who don't think you can achieve your dream body! That's enough to get you going, isn't it?*

"Do not wear high heels when you do this!" —VALÉRIE

Suck 'em in!

While washing the dishes or preparing food at the kitchen counter, remember to keep your abs contracted at all times.

"I also contract my abs each time I go through a door!" —VALÉRIE

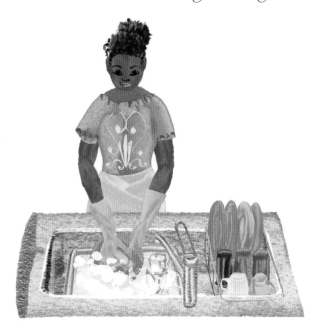

100-count squeeze

Sitting at a desk? In a movie theater? Make it count. An easy way to firm up your butt is to contract your bottom 100 times in a row. You can do a quick series and/or a slow series, holding the "squeeze" 3 seconds or longer each time. Do this exercise several times a day, and the result will be worthy of a thong!

DO IT NOW! *One way to remind yourself to squeeze those glutes: Wear something around your wrist, like a colorful bracelet. When you slip it on, tell yourself, "Each time I see this bracelet, I will do 50 glute contractions." The result? Over time, seeing the bracelet will automatically make you contract your glutes. You won't even have to think about it! How about doing a quick series of 100 right now?*

"If I'm in a place where someone might notice my body shifting as I do this, I substitute a single lon-n-n-ng squeeze instead. It usually lasts a minute, and, oh, does it burn!" —VALÉRIE

Pay attention to carbs

Refined carbs—white bread and pasta—go right to your waistline.
Complex ones, such as whole-grain breads, fuel your body.

GRAB & GO! *Keep a container of homemade hummus in the fridge. Then when a craving for something salty hits, you can grab a whole-grained cracker or even a baby carrot and dip — or just use your finger! (See my own personal recipe on page 142.)*

DO IT NOW! *Some "experts" suggest you tape a picture of yourself looking flabby and overweight on your fridge to discourage yourself from eating the "wrong" things. Instead, why not cut out a perfect-body photo from a magazine (beware, we are not talking about an out-of-reach Photoshopped skeletal body, but a healthy-looking toned one), put a photo cutout of your face on top and tape the result to your fridge. Now that's motivation!*

Sport your glutes!

The next time you attend a sporting event, focus on something that happens frequently during the game—a goal in basketball, a whistle in ice hockey, a penalty flag in football. Whenever it happens, squeeze your glutes and lift yourself up using the power of your arms. You'll not only tone your glutes but also build lovely biceps and triceps.

LE PETIT SECRET *Every time there's a time-out in the game you're watching, get up. But don't head for the refreshment stand. Instead, run up some stairs, jog around the stadium, walk fast around another level, then jog back downstairs.*

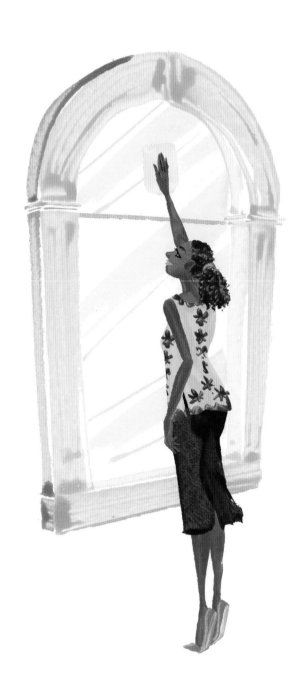

Clean 'til you're lean!

If you have cleaning people, give them a break and save some good money by doing the housework yourself, especially when it comes to the windows. It will work your cardio, build your flexibility, and help develop healthy shoulder joints. Remember to squat when you clean the lower portion of the windows—and to do calf raises when you clean the top parts!

DO IT NOW! *If you clean at a fast pace, in 1 hour you'll burn over 400 calories!*

LE PETIT SECRET *Studies show that laughter affects both mind and body. It lowers blood pressure and stress hormones, increases your pain threshold, boosts the immune system, and most important, with just 15 minutes of laughter, gives your lungs, abs, and heart the equivalent of a 15-minute cycling workout! So let go of your anger and negativity, enjoy life, and laugh at least 30 minutes a day. Watch a comedy, tell jokes to your friends, send them e-mail jokes. In short, have fun!*

Do the wave

If you're a baseball, football, or soccer fan, you probably spend a fair amount of time attending games. But just because you're not on the field doesn't mean you can just sit there. Instead, do the wave whenever it starts to move through the stands. It's an easy way to get moving while the game is on. Jump high, bring your arms up, and scream!

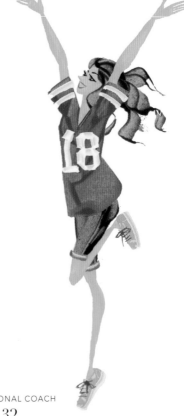

DO IT NOW! *If you lack the motivation to get moving, try this simple trick: Set your cell phone to ring every hour. Each time it rings, do something active. Go for a walk around the stadium or, when at home, take a walk around the block or do 15 jumping jacks. Do anything, but make sure you're moving!*

Work those stoplights

When you drive, each time you get to a red light, suck in your stomach during the entire duration of the light. Contract the lower abs for 5 seconds, release, then add the upper abs for another 5 seconds. Remember to breathe!

"If you can't find a way to laugh at yourself, then it's time to sign up for laughter classes! Don't laugh! These classes really do exist! If you don't believe me, just Google it!" —VALÉRIE

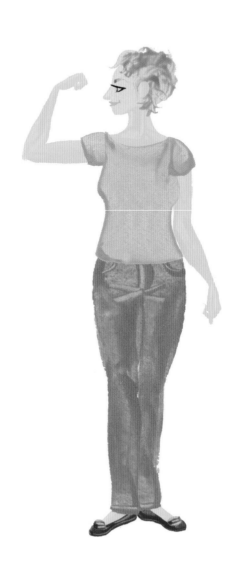

Strike a pose

If you have one minute, a mirror, and some privacy, strike a pose. Isolate a muscle group and flex it 10 times in a row. Hold each flex for 15 seconds. It won't take long to whip those muscles into shape!

LE PETIT SECRET *Wear fitted clothes. You can't motivate yourself to exercise if you hide your body under a pile of loose clothes. In fact, covering up with parachute-shaped clothes will make you gain weight. You'll lose touch with your real body size!*

DO IT NOW! *Watch yourself in store windows as you shop. Next time you do, you'll look fitter and trimer!*

"If I'm on a business trip and I have no time at all to tone and tighten after my shower, I make sure I at least do these flexes." —VALÉRIE

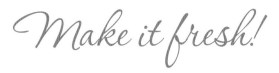

Make it fresh!

Eat fresh salads of raw vegetables regularly, along with your own homemade almond milk and fruit juices. (See page 141 for my fabulous Almond Milk recipe.) A former coach of mine at MyPrivateCoach, who has since become a best-selling recording artist, introduced me to the raw diet, and since then, with the help of my panel of nutritionists and dietitians, I have been avidly following the research being done on this subject.

In the end I discovered that I was not alone in having been successfully won over by the raw-food diet! In fact, Demi Moore owes her "youthfulness" not only to love and the (occasional) help of a scalpel but also to the benefits of raw foods. However, in her case, she became a 100 percent raw-diet aficionado before shooting *Charlie's Angels* and even had her own personal chef.

Sting is also a diehard "raw foodist" who admits owing his energy to a strict vegetarian diet. Woody Harrelson, Martina Navratilova, Madonna, Alicia Silverstone, Angela Bassett, and even Barbra Streisand follow, or have followed, a 75 to 100 percent all raw-vegetable diet.

Some doctors believe that adding more fresh vegetables to a diet does us good, and as such, they, too, have become supporters of the raw-food diet. Nonbelievers, on the other hand, argue that for a person not knowledgeable about nutrition, the hazards related to low levels of protein, amino acid, and iron deficiencies are pretty high. A 100 percent raw foodist may be in grave danger if he or she is not properly informed of the diet's pros and cons.

So, as usual, your coach reminds you that moderation is the way to go. If you like meat, dairy products, mashed potatoes, rice, and other cooked dishes, don't deprive yourself of these yummies! But keep an open mind and think about whether eating more fresh raw veggies is right for you. Aim for making raw food 50 percent of your diet, and you'll already be well on the road to a healthier and leaner you.

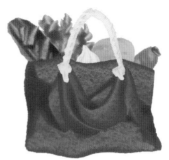

Take two

Take the stairs whenever the opportunity arises. And when you do, take them two at a time.

Concentrate on your form as you climb. Stand tall, tighten your abs, and don't lean forward too much. When you take the stairs two by two, you increase the load on the quadricep muscles in your thighs and the glutes in your butt. And that will add more definition and strength to both areas. Make sure you put your feet flat on the stairs to avoid getting bulgy calves!

"This is how French women get their lean, strong thighs. No elevators for us!" —VALÉRIE

DO IT NOW! *On days when it's hard to get moving, pinch your inner thighs so that their flabby cottage-cheese appearance is more obvious. One look should be all it takes to get yourself on track.*

No-sweat abs

Whenever you walk, contract your upper and lower abs at all times. This will help work the deep abdominal muscles that no crunches can reach. It will also help you create a flat stomach without any sweating at all!

QUICK TRICK!

Wear something around your wrist—a bracelet, watch, even an elastic band—as a reminder to hold in your abs during the day. You can also decide to "zip it up" each time you go through a door.

"Every time you carry a file or a book when you walk, hold the object as if you were hugging it. This will release the tension in your shoulder blades and make you feel more relaxed." —VALÉRIE

Sit on an invisible chair!

Lean your back flat against a wall with your feet shoulder-width apart—roughly 15 inches. Your heels should be approximately 12 to 16 inches from the wall. Now slide down the wall until you look as if you're sitting on an invisible chair. Your legs should be at a 90-degree angle when you stop.

Make sure your back is flat and your knees don't go over your toes; otherwise, you may create unnecessary pressure in your knee joints.

Hold this position for 1 minute. If you don't have the strength to hold the position that long, stand up and rest, then repeat. Keep repeating until you reach a total time of 1 minute for all your tries.

And lose the high heels before you attempt this!

"One of my invisible-chair champions is a bootcamper who just turned 78 last year. She can stay in this position for 10 minutes!" —VALÉRIE

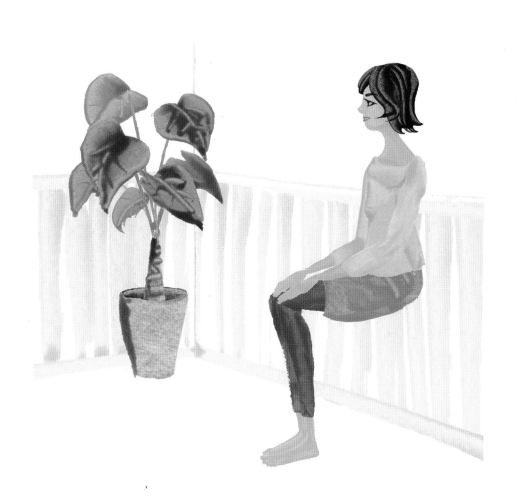

Take the day off

Is your coach losing her mind? Not quite. There are three situations where you should take the day off from exercise. Here's what they are:

- **When you don't feel well.** If you're feeling a little slumped because you're coming down with something, it's actually a message from your body saying, "I need to slow down because I need all my energy to get better, and please don't force me to use up that energy." This means no gym sessions, eating light meals, and no sugar intake (high glucose-level foods tend to put a strain on the immune system in the short term). Instead, eat lots of fresh fruit. Run a bath, read a book, get some rest, and let your body mend itself at its own pace.

- **When you haven't slept a wink.** Same story. Your body is exhausted. It needs to recharge its batteries. Eat light meals (as if you have a cold), but take tons of vitamins and a few short walks outdoors to replenish your body. Don't do anything more than that. DON'T go running full-speed on the treadmill and DO skip your samba class. You can do light yoga if it helps you recharge your emotional batteries.

- **When you're sick of working out or you're exhausted from yesterday's workout.** You deserve a rest! You can say, "I quit," but just for one day! Instead of working out, take this day to pamper yourself with a facial, a massage, some meditation, or some yoga, just to relax those achy muscles and soften those twisted joints. And on that note, I'm off to take a warm sudsy bath with lavender and sea salts. I need to relax my muscles after such a tense workout yesterday!

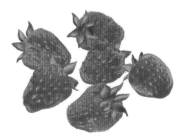

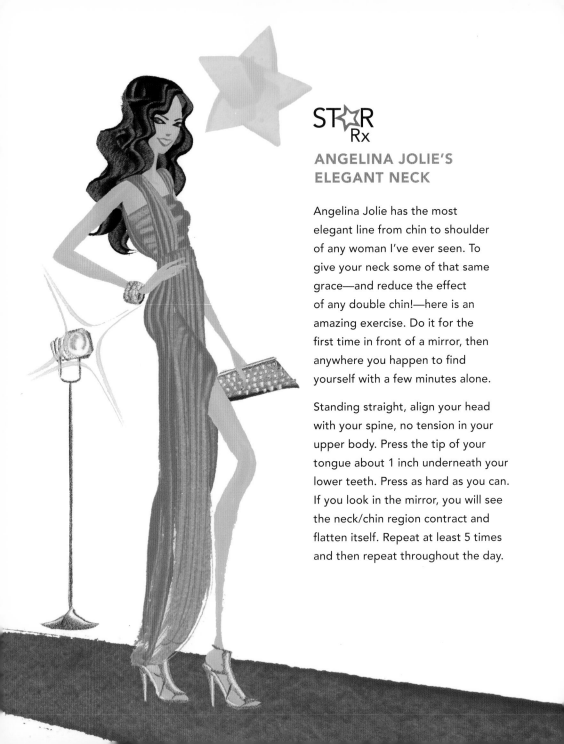

ST★R Rx

ANGELINA JOLIE'S ELEGANT NECK

Angelina Jolie has the most elegant line from chin to shoulder of any woman I've ever seen. To give your neck some of that same grace—and reduce the effect of any double chin!—here is an amazing exercise. Do it for the first time in front of a mirror, then anywhere you happen to find yourself with a few minutes alone.

Standing straight, align your head with your spine, no tension in your upper body. Press the tip of your tongue about 1 inch underneath your lower teeth. Press as hard as you can. If you look in the mirror, you will see the neck/chin region contract and flatten itself. Repeat at least 5 times and then repeat throughout the day.

Play with your posture

Perfect posture is what gives many film stars, celebrities, and even royalty that lovely line and elegance that frequently sets them apart. To perfect your posture, find a wall and stand with your back, butt, and heels against it. (If you're wearing high-heeled shoes, please remove them first.) Pull your shoulders back so that they're against the wall, too.

Now, with your heels, butt, back, and shoulders all against the wall, raise your arms slowly in front of you until they're straight above your head. Don't arch your back. Try to touch your thumbs to the wall above your head.

Breathe out as you raise your arms. Breathe in as you lower them.

Do this exercise 15 times, rest for a minute, and repeat the entire set.

Repeat this sequence at least 3 times throughout the day. At first it might sound impossible to do this exercise without arching your back, but the more you repeat it, the better you will become.

Run the airport racetrack

If you arrive at the airport at least 90 minutes before departure, you'll be less stressed about missing your flight, you'll probably clear security faster, and you'll have plenty of time to walk those mile-long halls to your gate—a couple of times!

QUICK TRICK!

To learn how to differentiate your lower, middle, and upper abs, look at yourself in a mirror with your abs uncovered. Suck in your lower abs, then watch in the mirror as you sequentially move up to first your middle abs and then your upper abs. Once you've visually isolated each muscle group, working on lower/upper abs will be easy.

LE PETIT SECRET *Wear a pedometer at the airport and aim to walk 5,000 steps. Don't sit until you've reached your goal. If you have a small child, push the stroller. It will add some nice tone to your arms!*

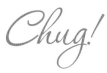

Chug!

A 1 percent decrease in your level of hydration triggers a loss of energy and a discernible level of fatigue. Your mood tends to oscillate. This is followed by a total disinterest in what your favorite coach (me) is teaching you. You don't want to run, walk, dance, or do much. You may also feel sluggish and lazy.

The worst thing you can do in this situation is to drown your sorrows in a steaming cup of hot coffee or a soda. Both dehydrate your body, as does black tea and alcohol.

Instead, drink water, sparkling water, green or white tea, vegetable juice, milk, even fruit juice. All will bring your hydration levels back up so you'll feel full of energy and ready to squeeze some glutes!

GRAB & GO! *Keep your fridge, workplace, and car stocked with bottled water or green tea to stay hydrated. Avoid diet sodas. Studies show they make you eat more. Plus, they trigger a blood-sugar response that encourages your body to store fat.*

DO IT NOW! *Need more motivation to keep moving? Put your weight-loss curve on the fridge. You can't miss it. And it makes you more accountable to yourself.*

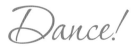

Dance!

Whenever you're working at home, stand up, turn on your favorite fast-paced music, and dance. Nobody's there but you, so let go of your toxic thoughts and stress. You can jump, swirl, and jump again! Get crazy! Do it every hour.

DO IT NOW! *If you dance 6 times a day, that's 20 minutes of cardio!*

"My favorite music to dance to?
'Will Survive!'" —VALERIE

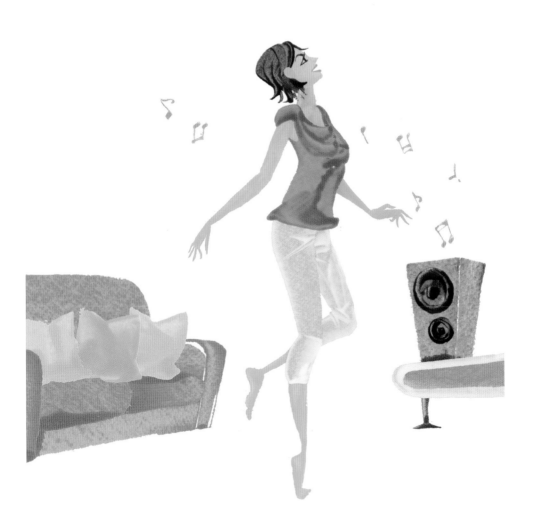

Sneaker TV

Make sure you're wearing sneakers when you turn on the TV.
When commercials start, jump to your feet, switch the channel to
any exercise station, and work out until your program resumes. If
you're not into fitness TV, then do 50 jumping jacks. They'll not
only burn calories, they'll increase your bone density as well.

DO IT NOW! *Revenge is a great motivator.*
Your boyfriend dumped you? You'll show him who
the hottest chick on the planet is! Tape a picture
of him to the fridge to jump-start your day.

Lift and relax

Working on a computer can create a lot of stress on your
shoulders and neck. Here's a quick fix: Lift your shoulders as close
to your ears as possible. Hold for 5 seconds, then relax. Repeat
10 times and you'll look as great as you feel.

Watch the soaps

The average American watches nearly 3 hours of TV a day. But if you have a stationary bike, an elliptical strider, a mini peddler, or a mini stepper (you can get one for under $40), you can also use that time to burn calories. So click on your favorite soap—or even slip a movie into the DVD player—and start to move. Just pick a pace and hold it. By watching an interesting show or movie, you'll take your mind off the effort it takes to peddle or step—and you'll probably do more than you otherwise would!

"One added benefit of exercising while watching TV: It'll take your mind off the snacks and other fattening foods you might otherwise eat while watching!" —VALÉRIE

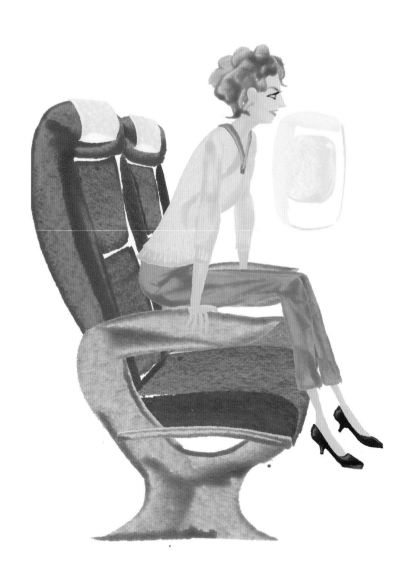

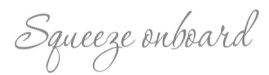

Squeeze onboard

Flying to Paris? Aruba? Montreal? Your mom's? Whenever you're onboard an aircraft, do a series of 25 slow glute squeezes every hour. Finish each series with a stronger squeeze; hold for 5 seconds. Go for the burn! Follow this with a series of 10 lower ab contractions. Finish with a long ab squeeze of at least 20 seconds. Repeat the same exercise with your upper abs. Here are three other moves:

- **Tone your thighs while seated.** Raise up your knees, keeping a 90-degree angle between your thighs and calves. Lower your knees. Repeat 100 times, slowly, maintaining control of your move at all times. As an extra bonus, keep your abs tight during this exercise.

- **Get strong arms.** Using your armrests, lift yourself up using only your arm strength. Hold each lift for a count of 5. Repeat 4 times.

- **Stretch your legs as straight and high as you can.** Hold for 5 seconds. Then, keeping your legs lifted, lean forward, keeping your back straight. This will stretch the backs of your thighs and your lower back.

Drive the bulge away

When driving long distances, stop every hour. Drink plain water—not icy, just room temperature—or caffeine-free green tea. Walk for 5 to 7 minutes to get your heart pumping and your body oxygenated. Then do 50 jumping jacks before you jump back in the car.

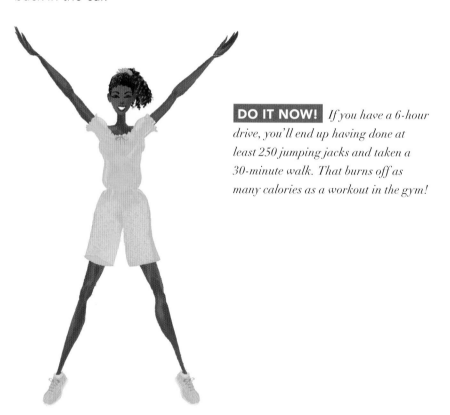

DO IT NOW! *If you have a 6-hour drive, you'll end up having done at least 250 jumping jacks and taken a 30-minute walk. That burns off as many calories as a workout in the gym!*

By all means, fidget

Remember your mom saying, "Stop fidgeting!" Well, don't listen to her anymore. Even fidgeting in your seat burns calories—in fact, it burns twice as many calories as just sitting or standing. So feel free to fidget and wiggle around constantly—at your desk, in a line, even waiting for a stoplight!

"I am a professional fidgeter myself! And now that I know it's totally legit, I fidget waiting in line everywhere—at the movies, at the supermarket, in the airport. I even teach fidgeting to my friends!" —VALÉRIE

Zip—unzip!

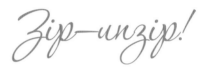

Here's a fast way to increase your range of motion and keep your shoulders loose and flexible. Several times a day, pretend you're zipping and unzipping a dress with a back zipper. With one hand, start from the bottom and "zip up" as far as you can between your shoulder blades. Finish by taking the other arm and reaching down over your shoulder and pulling the "zipper" up farther. Then reverse hands and repeat.

"I do this in an elevator—when I'm alone!" —VALÉRIE

. . . .

Ditch the waiting room

The next time you drop off your kids at the dentist, don't sit in the waiting room. Instead, go for a walk. A cleaning usually lasts 30 minutes, and a cavity treatment lasts an hour.

DO IT NOW! *Studies reveal that the path to good health is built with 10,000 steps a day. So always wear a pedometer wherever you go, and check the readout whenever you have a free minute. If it's not over 10,000, get up and walk somewhere!*

Can some lifts

Take two large cans—two 2-pound (907-g) cans of tomato sauce are perfect—and stand straight with your knees slightly bent. Tuck in your stomach, then place your elbows against your rib cage so that you use only your bicep power. Do alternate raises while looking at the muscle that's contracting. Aim at achieving a series of 15 raises for each arm. Do 4 reps, pausing in between.

QUICK TRICK!

Want the backs of your arms to have curves rather than flab? If you are carrying groceries and have a heavy package in your bag—8 to 10 pounds is perfect—hold it with both hands and do 15 French curls. Stand straight, feet shoulder-width apart, stomach and back flat, and lift your arms over your head.

"The triceps muscle on the back of your arms is hard to sculpt. But it's important to firm it up if you want to look good in a sleeveless top." —VALÉRIE

Squeeze and fold

Take advantage of the time you spend doing laundry!
Whenever you fold laundry, use the time to squeeze your glutes as fast as you can. Nobody will see you, so don't be afraid of looking ridiculous! By squeezing as you fold, you'll quite literally squeeze some necessary toning exercises into your busy day. And the more laundry you do, the more toned your curves will be!

DO IT NOW! *Get yourself some support. Visit a forum like the ones at my weight-loss website LeBootCamp.com. Or create your own, made up of friends and colleagues. The support will motivate you to stay on track. Go online for 5 minutes in the morning and 5 minutes at night. You'll get a lot of support, and you'll give a lot as well. And—of course!— contract your glutes and abs as long as you stay online!*

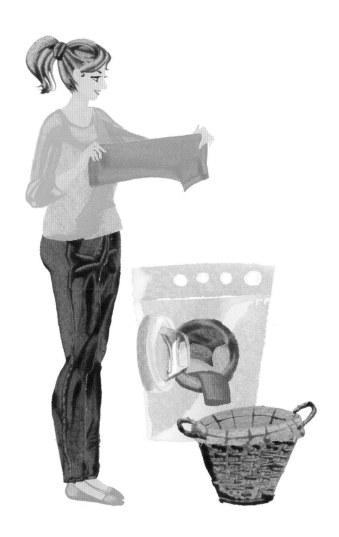

The Security Squeeze

At the airport don't stand around endlessly, dreading the fact that you will have to remove your shoes in front of hundreds of people. Instead, use the time at airport security checkpoints to squeeze your glutes. Nobody will notice. And with the typical wait, you'll get up to 300 squeezes before you head toward your gate. If you want to keep your squeezes discreet, simply shift your body weight from one leg to the other, alternating cheek squeezes.

"Since I travel a lot, I apply these tips at airports frequently. And with the long lines at security checkpoints, I tend to squeeze, and squeeze, and squeeze." —VALÉRIE

Work it!

When you're working alone or with friends in the kitchen, put on some music and dance. I did it just last night to burn off a few extra calories that were sneaking into my sauce. I listened to Katy Perry, Muse ("Supermassive Black Hole"), Lady Gaga, and Lady Antebellum while I set the table and whipped up a wonderful dinner. I'd set a plate on the table, then do a few steps, move to the next place setting, set down a plate, do a few steps, and move on. Even while stirring a sauce on the stove, I'd move my hips in the same direction I was stirring the sauce in my saucepan!

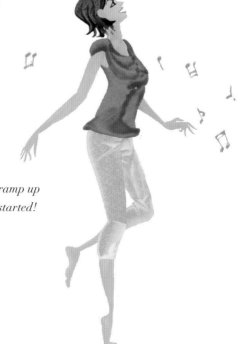

DO IT NOW! *This is a great way to ramp up the mood of a party when it's just getting started!*

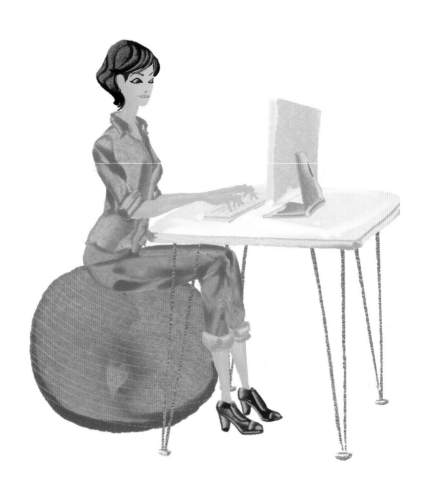

Have a ball while you sit

If you sit at a desk all day, replace your chair with a stability ball—one of those huge balls almost as big as a chair. Prolonged sitting weakens the spine, but because the stability ball moves whenever you do—forcing you to work your abdominals and work on your balance—it actually strengthens the muscles that support your spine.

QUICK TRICK!

Every hour or so, stretch out on the ball. Lie with your back across the top of the ball, and roll the ball back and forth a few inches by pressing your feet into the floor. And if you're sitting at your desk on a ball and no one's around, bounce up and down as long as you can. This trick will pick up your blood and lymph circulation. Besides, you'll have a blast!

"If stress rules your life, open a window and breathe some fresh air as soon as you wake up. Breathe in deeply through your nose, feeling the air swell your abdomen and chest. Hold for a count of 5, then slowly exhale." —VALÉRIE

Walk and squeeze

When you walk, with each step squeeze the side of your derriere on your back leg. A strong squeeze! This is a very, very French exercise. My mom, my mother-in-law . . . all the women I know in France use this simple trick.

DO IT NOW! *Consistently squeezing glutes can give you a sexy walk within one single month!*

Wear a vest

Buy yourself a weight vest at a sports store, load it with 10 to 15 pounds of weights, and walk for 30 minutes. Or better yet, borrow your dad's fishing vest, load it with rocks, and head out for a stroll!

DO IT NOW! *You'll burn 180 calories more than you normally would on a 30-minute walk!*

ST☆R Rx

GISELE BÜNDCHEN'S RACY BACK

A flabby back is pretty unsightly in a summer dress or bathing suit. However, because we don't get to see our own backs, we tend to forget about toning this hidden body part. Here's an easy, fast way to get a nicely defined back like Brazilian model Gisele Bündchen:

1. When watching TV, take two 5-pound (2.27-kg) dumbbells, one in each hand. Sit comfortably, keep your back straight, and bend at hip level so that your breasts almost touch your knees.

2. Start with your dumbbells touching the floor and slowly sit up, keeping your arms as close to your trunk as possible until your hands are at breast level. Go back down immediately. Do this move as slowly as possible. Repeat until it burns. When finished, hug yourself to stretch the muscles you just worked on.

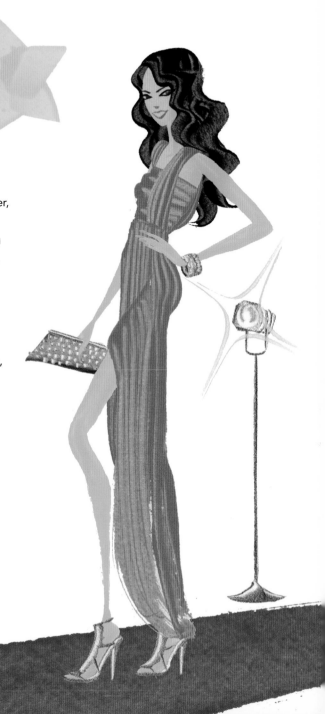

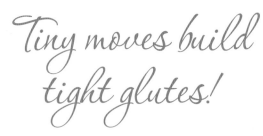

Tiny moves build tight glutes!

Waiting at another crosswalk? Try something new. Stand straight and put almost all your weight on one leg. Swing the other leg back behind the first until you feel a squeeze in your glutes. Touch your toes to the ground, then swing the leg forward until it's where you started.

Go back and forth with this small move until it burns, then switch legs and stand on the one you originally had behind you.

"If you don't have time to exercise both legs, remember to start at the next crosswalk with the leg you missed!" —VALÉRIE

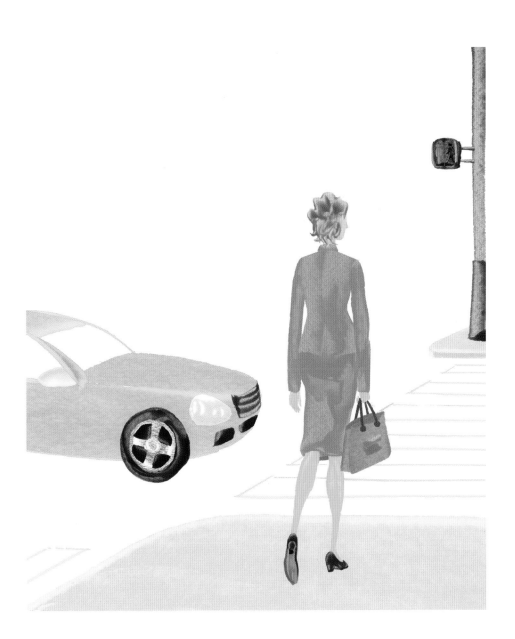

Say good-bye to love handles

All it takes to lose those love handles is 5 minutes a day. You can even do it in your workplace. Here's how:

Sit in the center of a chair with your feet resting flat on the floor. You must sit comfortably and have the entire length of your thighs resting on the chair.

Grab a book, a bottle, or anything that you can handle with two hands and weighs just a couple of pounds. Keep your back straight and your abs tight but not totally sucked in. Lift the object you're holding to breast level and slowly rotate your upper body at waist level from right to left and from left to right. Your head should follow the move. Hold the position on each side of the rotation for a count of 2—or until your boss pops in!

Start with a light weight, then slowly increase the weight and time as you feel more comfortable with the move. Work your way up to 2 minutes in the morning and 3 minutes in the afternoon.

The popcorn alternative

When you slip a disc into the DVD player and settle down to watch a movie, keep your hands busy with a couple of weights instead of the popcorn bowl. Pick up two 5-pound (2.27-g) dumbbells and do a few bicep curls.

You can do this either sitting or standing with your back and stomach tight. Keep your elbows as close to your rib cage as possible, and lift each weight up and down. Alternate sides. Do not let your muscles rest during the repetition. Aim for 15 reps. Repeat until you can't possibly continue. Then add 5 more!

"If you're really craving popcorn, measure out a single cup and eat it as you pedal a stationary bike. Stop eating as soon as you stop pedaling!" —VALÉRIE

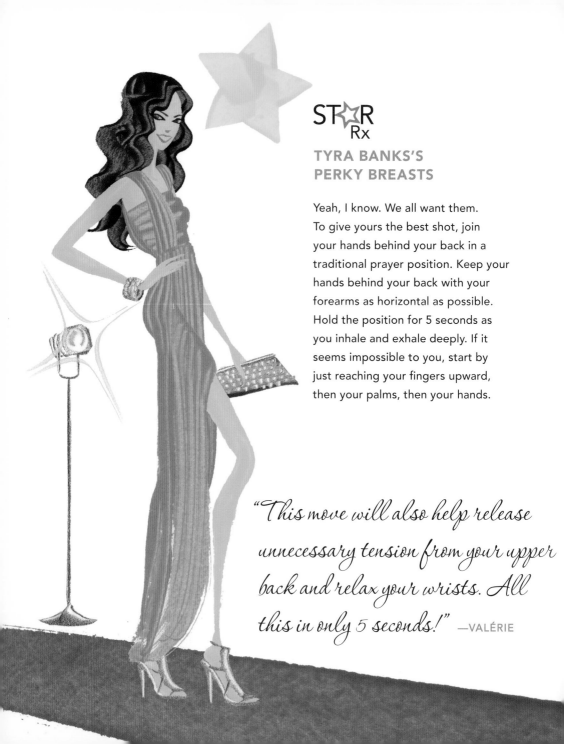

ST☆R Rx

TYRA BANKS'S PERKY BREASTS

Yeah, I know. We all want them. To give yours the best shot, join your hands behind your back in a traditional prayer position. Keep your hands behind your back with your forearms as horizontal as possible. Hold the position for 5 seconds as you inhale and exhale deeply. If it seems impossible to you, start by just reaching your fingers upward, then your palms, then your hands.

"This move will also help release unnecessary tension from your upper back and relax your wrists. All this in only 5 seconds!" —VALÉRIE

Plant a garden

Every time you spend an hour planting, watering, and weeding, you get an amazing burst of endorphins—the hormones of happiness. And when you're happy, you are less hungry.

DO IT NOW! *An hour's worth of garden work can burn 300 calories!*

. . . .

Pick it yourself

There are more and more farms that open their fields to customers willing to pick their own fruits and vegetables. Give it a try. Take your whole family—the kids will love it—and you'll all get lots of great exercise.

LE PETIT SECRET *Freshly picked fruits and vegetables have peak levels of antioxidants and nutrients.*

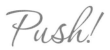

Push!

Use a push mower to mow your lawn instead of a power mower. Not only will you save money (just calculate how much this will save in a year!), but if you use a push mower, you will also "spend" 400 calories an hour—100 calories more than if you used a power mower.

"Taking care of gardens and lawns is essential for your well-being. Being in contact with nature is important for a balanced life." —VALÉRIE

DO IT NOW! *Getting enough natural light will help you sleep. So put down this book, head outdoors, and mow!*

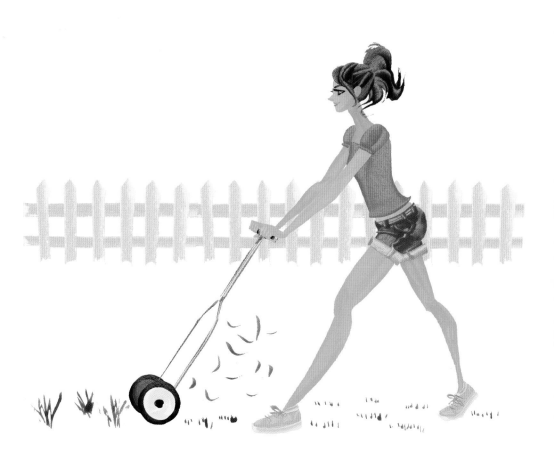

Move the recycling bins

Place the recycling bins as far away from your workstation as possible. This will force you to stand up and move every time you need to throw something away. When you stand up, use the full power of your thighs to stand (as slow as you can without looking sick to your colleagues), and walk to the bin and back. Those little extra moves can represent 2 pounds of fat lost per year without having to change anything in your diet or even your gym routine.

"And don't try to play basketball with the bin. I'm sure you might be tempted!" —VALÉRIE

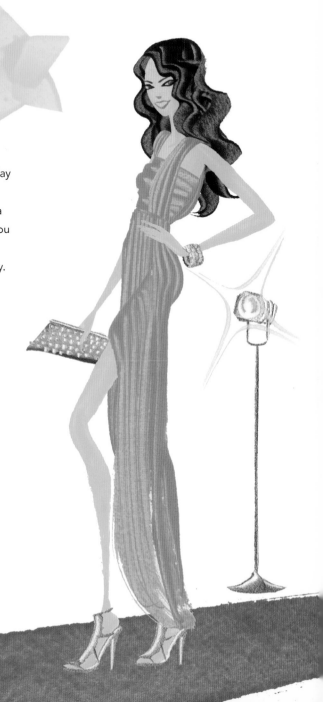

STⒶR
Rx

KIM KARDASHIAN'S FIRM BOOTY

Kim is a woman who knows how to play with her curves. She is not ashamed of being curvy and being more than a size 0 or 2—and she is proving that you can have curves without being hit by gravity. Her butt is firm but not flabby.

A killer quickie move to get a steel booty like Kim's is the one-legged squat with a Swiss ball. I leave a Swiss ball in my living room and each time I walk past it, I do the following exercise 20 times:

With the ball against the wall, stand with a straight back against the ball. Squat on one leg, pushing as much as you can on the ball to balance your body and, using the power of your booty, raise yourself back up. It should burn. Make sure the knee that you bend is pointing outward to avoid putting too much pressure on your joint. I never do more than 20 at a time.

Eat wisely before you pig out!

If you have a business dinner scheduled, and you know the menu is going to have piles of everything that makes you fat— steak, dips, alcohol, cake—two tricks will help you avoid the inevitable. One, the day before your dinner, eat very lightly. Opt for cold soups, like gazpacho, and a rich salad full of seasonal veggies but light on the dressing. And two, on the day of your dinner, eat lightly and have a bite or two of appetite-killing protein—a hard-boiled egg is perfect—on the way to the dinner.

LE PETIT SECRET *A number of French women wear a ribbon around their waist and underneath their clothes when they go out to dinner. It keeps them conscious of the tummy— particularly if the ribbon starts to feel tighter as the evening goes on!*

Ball game, anyone?

Instead of just stuffing yourself at the neighborhood barbecue, bring a soccer ball and play with your friends. A soccer game uses up 400 calories an hour! That's enough to cover that big piece of meat you're about to enjoy!

If your barbecue is on a beach, then opt for beach volleyball. You'll burn 500 calories, work your cardio, and—with all that jumping!—build bone density.

"Coach's orders: Always have a ball in your car trunk!" —VALÉRIE

DO IT NOW! *Challenge your neighbors to see how many different kinds of vegetables they can put into whatever dish they're bringing to the barbecue. Try to reach a goal of 100 veggies for the neighborhood. When you add in the spices on everything or when you count the different varieties of a vegetable like potatoes, it's not as hard as it seems!*

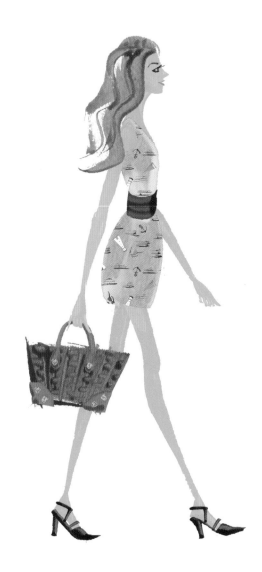

End your double chin

While you're shedding those extra annoying pounds, you may still suffer from a double chin. The extra chin isn't very elegant—and it should disappear if you follow this book's advice. But until it does, here's a secret to make it disappear: Walk like a queen. Keep your back straight, head over your shoulders, look straight ahead, and pull your chin forward.

We tend to have a sloppy posture that makes a double chin more prominent. If you walk as straight as you can and keep your head up, you will greatly reduce this disgraceful extra "skin."

"This may not seem too comfortable at first, because we're used to walking with our heads down. But persevere. After a few weeks, chances are, your friends will ask if you've lost weight before you actually start losing weight for real!" —VALÉRIE

Breastfeed your baby

Making all that milk will burn 500 calories a day! You'll be out of your "preggy" pants and into a pair of slim jeans in no time!

DO IT NOW! *Breastfeeding is the most amazing way to begin a close relationship with your son or daughter—one that will last a lifetime.*

. . . .

The 3-second butt builder

Each time you go to sit, stand back up before your butt actually hits the chair. Just do it once each time. The average person who works in an office stands up and sits back down on a chair at least 50 times a day. That's 50 squats. And each one only takes 3 seconds!

The 2-minute refresher

If you work at a desk and are constantly looking at a screen, chances are that your eyes are tense.

You may even be squinting—not a good thing when you want to prevent lines.

To avoid them, periodically close your eyes, relax your entire face, and place your palms over your eyes. Apply gentle pressure. Breathe deeply.

QUICK TRICK!

To relieve tension, try this 2-minute exercise: Sit comfortably, back straight, and gently put your hands on your thighs. Inhale deeply. Feel your abdomen swell and your chest fill with fresh air. Hold for 2 seconds. Exhale as strongly as you can, saying, "Ha!" (if you don't have colleagues who might make fun of you).

Now move your palms from your eyes to your cheeks and press again. Remember to let your entire face relax. After 30 seconds move your palms to your temples. Breathe.

In only 2 minutes you'll feel refreshed and ready to go. Repeat this exercise each time you feel tension building in your body. Once an hour should keep your eye area tension-free.

Raise your knees

When you're just sitting around, raise first one knee, then another for a full minute. Repeat every time you move to a new chair or couch.

"Invent your own mantra that will kick you in the butt when your butt feels like staying on the couch. Repeat every time you find yourself just lying around. My own mantra is, 'Trying is not enough; you've got to succeed.' I repeat it so much, it's now become part of who I am." —VALÉRIE

ST★R Rx

HALLE BERRY'S SEXY THIGHS

Remember seeing Halle Berry coming out of the water in *Die Another Day*? Want the same thighs? It's possible!

Ride your bike to and from work. If you work too far away, then find a way to swim 3 times a week at lunchtime. If you can't do either, then do squats while brushing your teeth. With feet 1 foot apart, back straight, and 1 hand on the sink, slowly squat down until knees are at a 90-degree angle, then come back up.

Or do the sumo crab walk when home alone. (I do this one while putting the laundry away.) Here's how:

1. Get into a sumo wrestling stance: your feet wider than shoulder-width apart, toes pointed out, and knees extended over the toes.

2. Keep your back straight, chest out, and abs tight throughout this move.

3. In this almost-sitting position, take a step forward, one foot at a time.

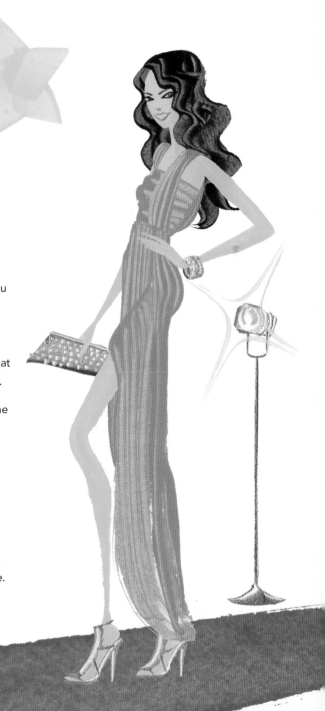

Encourage your friends

Share these tips with friends and, together, make a commitment to achieve a fabulous body. Sharing goals is one of the best ways to achieve them, since it increases our feeling of commitment.

LE PETIT SECRET *Fake friends are energy vampires! Get rid of all the people who tell you, "You won't make it," "It's your twelfth diet; you are doomed," "I brought some carrot cake for your afternoon snack," or "How about we enjoy an ice cream instead of going to the gym?" Avoid interacting with these saboteurs until you've reached a few milestones that will guarantee you never turn back to where you were before. Granted, in the 21st century it's harder to clean up your address book since you need to go through all those social networking sites, through your e-mail address book, your cell phone, etc. . . . but it's worth your time.*

Be a stair master

If you have stairs at home, use them. Make it a habit to climb them as fast as you can several times a day. If you need a purpose, find something—laundry, for example—that needs to be carried up or down. Then do it one piece at a time.

QUICK TRICK!

Stairs are everywhere, so why not make them a part of your everyday exercise program? Climbing stairs helps build nice legs as well as a firm rear. Remember to keep your stomach tucked in.

"Be sure to put your feet flat on the stairs to avoid building oversized calves." —VALÉRIE

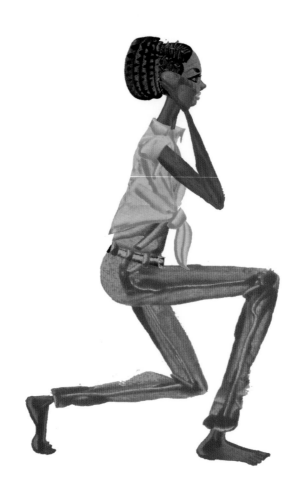

Phone lunges

You already know that you can walk and squeeze your glutes when you're on the phone. Now try something harder: Whenever you talk with a friend or family member—or anyone else who won't be alarmed by your huffing and puffing—lunge forward. And not just once. Do it continuously for the whole length of your call. A daily 10-minute call peppered with lunges will help shape your thighs and strengthen the bottom part of your glutes—which makes you look nicer in a bathing suit!

QUICK TRICK!

Sometimes I do phone lunges and climb stairs at home while I'm talking with my mom. She thinks I'm out of shape because I'm huffing and puffing as we talk. Little does she know I'm simply climbing the stairs two at a time while talking—or, more likely, listening—to her!

"If I'm on the phone for a long time, I spike my lunges with the occasional jumping jack just to keep things interesting." —VALÉRIE

Work while your kids play

Don't just stand around talking with other moms while your kids are playing with their friends on the playground. Instead, start a playground workout parent group so you can all get the exercise moms need. You can keep an eye on the kids while they swing—and burn some calories at the same time.

Start by walking around the playground or play-area perimeter. Try to walk for at least 15 minutes, preferably 30. Once you're warmed up, locate a picnic bench (there's always one around somewhere!) or anything that can be used as a high step. Now do 5 steps-ups on the same leg and make a particularly strong push for the last step. Repeat with the other leg. Make sure you put your foot flat to avoid inflating your calves and to isolate the move in your glutes and thighs. Then do 20 jumping jacks. Repeat step-ups with 10 reps per leg. Do 20 more jumping jacks and repeat step-ups with 15 reps per leg.

At this point you should feel a burn in your muscles. That signals it's time to return to your kids on the slide! One caveat: If you turn your attention away from the kids for even a second, make sure one of the other moms is watching them. Then you can return the favor!

Practice toilet squats

If you drink the 10 glasses of water a day most doctors advise, chances are that you'll spend a lot of time in the bathroom. Rather than looking at those bathroom breaks as a waste of time, however, you can use them to help build stronger and better-defined thighs. How? Instead of sitting on the toilet seat (where you don't know who sat before you, anyway!), squat over the seat to do your business. Stay in the squat until your business is finished. If you do this just 6 times a day, you're guaranteed great thighs for bathing-suit season!

"Whoever would have thought that you could accomplish so much in the bathroom?" —VALÉRIE

DO IT NOW! *Feeling the burn that those toilet squats cause just might make you think twice about jumping into a vat of ice cream later in the day. You won't want them to have been in vain!*

Carry the kids

If you're attending a sporting event with your baby or small kids, carry them around as much as possible. Not only will they love being shown around by Mom, but adding weight on your shoulders and arms will also add strength.

. . . .

Halve your calves

In the unlikely event that you suffer from flabby calves, here's an easy exercise: Each time you stand up from a chair, bend your leg at the knee, raise your calf, and squeeze it as hard as you can for 2 seconds. If you do it each time you stand, you're guaranteed to get nicely shaped calves within a month or two. Keep it up!

Barbecue bun burner

Barbecues usually have a lot of kids running around, which many adults are not happy about, because all that exploding energy is making them dizzy! Kill four birds with one stone: Organize a run-hide-and-seek game with the kids, in which you participate, and you will:

- Burn extra calories.

- Make the kids happy.

- Make the adults happy.

- Eat less, since you will be far away from the food table.

This is an easy one, yes?

LE PETIT SECRET *Run around with those kids for two hours and you'll be able to burn off a hamburger and small fries!*

Shop at your local farmers market

A study in Spain found that those who shopped at a farmers market weighed 30 percent less than those who shopped at grocery stores.

Is it that only thin people buy their vegetables at the market? I don't think so!

My theory is that when you take the time to choose your fruits and veggies and put effort into your shopping, you actually take better care of yourself and become more aware of what is good for your body—no perfect-looking veggies (possibly genetically modified) in plastic packaging for you! Going to a farmers market obviously supports your local community, but it also creates the simple joy of being able to touch what you buy.

Purchasing your produce at the market will also help you stay in tune with the seasons. As a weight-loss coach, I believe that eating what nature offers at specific times during the year makes more sense than eating cherries in winter or pumpkins in summer.

Moreover, fruits and vegetables in season are grown and picked locally. Therefore, they reach your merchant faster and are packed with vitamins. This is not true with the veggies and fruits that sit in supermarkets for days, weeks, and sometimes even longer! Some of these are transported by plane or harvested when unripe and ripened in warehouses, or even if collected ripe, may take quite some time before landing in your kitchen.

And there's more! To get to the market, you will probably walk, while contracting your glutes and abs, of course, and you will interact with people when you go to a farmers market (much more than at the local supermarket), which makes the social aspect of the market fun, too. Enjoy the outdoors, enjoy touching what you buy, testing and tasting, meeting new people. Enjoy life!

On that note, I'm off to the market to buy some beautiful, ripe, vitamin-rich apples!

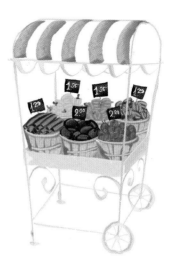

Jump for joy

When your team scores during a sporting event, joyfully jump as high as you can. Contract your thighs and calves, throw your arms high, jump, and just let yourself go. Scream as loud as you can. Screaming will help re-oxygenate you, while jumping builds bone and burns up calories.

"I'm a big sports fan myself. And when one of my teams is on a winning streak, I'll probably burn off 10,000 calories during the season!" —VALÉRIE

DO IT NOW! *You can even do this at home, watching with your family. They'll probably jump right along with you!*

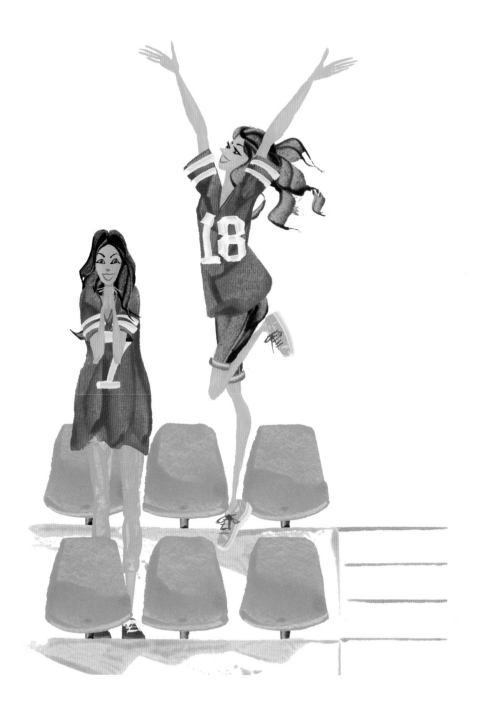

Pitch in!

Next time your neighbor invites you to a barbecue, help her out as much as you can. Help set the table, help clear up, help carry food and drinks. Do it for an hour and this light activity will help you burn the equivalent of one small soda.

And here's how to help yourself to more toned muscles while you help her.

- When you carry something, try to carry it with your arms extended in front of you to build a stronger upper body.

- If you have two bags of equal weight to carry, lift them with your biceps (forearms) instead of just having the bags drape over your wrists.

- When carrying cans and bottles, hold them like dumbbells and alternately bend your elbows and raise them using your biceps.

- Carry charcoal for the barbecue over your head to get lean, strong shoulders!

Get sold on cold

During the cold-weather season, turn your home thermostat as low as you can stand it when you're home. Then, every time you get cold, stand up and do 50 jumping jacks, a few squats, and a few arm swings. You'll end up burning calories every 20 minutes or so!

This easy tip will keep your blood flowing, shape your body, help keep your energy bill down, and let you be a true friend to the environment.

"In San Francisco, where I live, winters are not like in Wisconsin. But I still keep the temperature around 63°F in my house, which forces me to stand up often to do a few jumping jacks." —VALÉRIE

Ban drive-thrus from the planet

Have you noticed how many things you do every day at a drive-thru?

We are spending so much time in sedentary jobs that never having to physically mail a letter, get cash at the bank, buy food, or pick up a prescription refill is going to completely transform us into fossils. So avoid using these "convenient" drive-thrus! Totally!

Instead, park two blocks away, admire the sky, look at the trees lining the streets, walk to the bank, squeeze your glutes while waiting in line, walk to the post office, and smile at people on the street. And buy good, healthy food in a supermarket rather than zipping through a fast-food drive-thru! You will be healthier—therefore, requiring fewer prescriptions!

DO IT NOW! *By quitting your drive-thru habit, you can end up burning 350 more calories a week—which will turn into a 1-pound weight loss every 10 weeks! Isn't the healthy life beautiful?*

Add a few pounds

Add a few pounds to your normal body weight to burn more energy doing regular things throughout the day. Wear ankle weights under your pants (nobody will see them), wear a heavy backpack when walking, wear wrist weights under long sleeves as you shop for groceries. It's easy and it's fun!

....

Pick up the rake

If you're like a gazillion others who own a yard, chances are you hire someone else to rake all the unsightly leaves every fall. Well, stop right there! You're wasting your money and your health! Raking dead leaves burns 300 calories an hour!

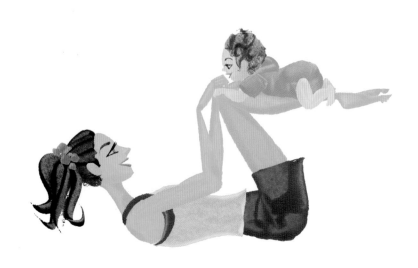

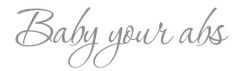
Baby your abs

A good way to get a nice flat stomach after pregnancy is to work on your abs several times a day. Get your doctor's approval first. Then, when you're in a comfortable environment, lie down with your baby on your chest in a comfy mom-baby position. Keeping your legs bent, lift your upper body for a count of 2. Your baby will add a nice weight to the exercise. Aim for 20 reps. And repeat as often as you can during the day.

DO IT NOW! *This is a great way to have fun with your baby! He or she will be happy to listen to your heart while you do this quick routine. However, always keep your baby's safety in mind when you are exercising together.*

Squat in the kitchen

Emptying the dishwasher? Squat down instead of bending. You'll end up doing at least 15 squats!

"This is why French women have such sexy derrières!" —VALÉRIE

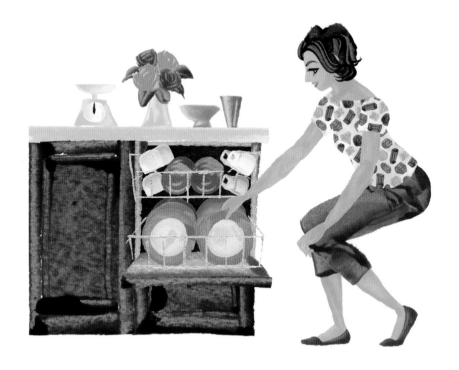

Fill 'er up!

Do you realize how long it takes to fill your gas tank? Anywhere between 3 and 7 minutes! So how about using those minutes to get fit? Here are my suggestions:

- Wash your windshield as fast as you can.

- Shift your weight from one leg to the other and squeeze your glutes each time you change sides.

- Empty all that trash out of the backseat!

- Rotate. No need to go wild—just spread your arms out, keep your hips straight, and twist your upper body to the left and right. If you do this every time you visit a gas station, you'll achieve a toned body without having to sweat for it.

DO IT NOW! *If you have a curb near your car, you can also go up and down the curb until the tank fills. (My fave!)*

Lunch on pomegranates

Pomegranate juice is everywhere today. But it's the skin that's loaded with powerful antioxidants called polyphenols, which may inhibit atherosclerosis, reduce the risk of cardiovascular diseases, and lower blood pressure. Buy the fruit when it's in season, and eat it raw or cooked with a touch of butter. The seeds are wonderful—sprinkle some on a slice of whole-grained toast smeared with hummus. Or enjoy the seeds sprinkled on fresh pineapple as a refreshing and antioxidant-loaded dessert. Yum!

"You don't need to spend money on sugary pomegranate juice or pricey supplements that claim to contain an extract of pomegranate skin. The whole fruit is fabulous all on its own." —VALÉRIE

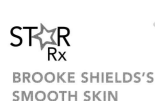

BROOKE SHIELDS'S
SMOOTH SKIN

Removing wrinkles is always painful (think "injections"), expensive, and hazardous to your overall face (think "unsuccessful face lift").

One of the best ways to stay wrinkle-free, apart from staying out of the sun, getting a good night's sleep, and not smoking, is to avoid creating what we call mechanical wrinkles (the ones linked to our facial expressions).

When I was a teenager, I remember reading an article where Brooke Shields said that to avoid forming wrinkles, she never, ever frowned while exercising. I was 16 when I read this, but I've kept her advice in mind ever since. So I pass it on to you: Do not frown when exercising. You don't need it, n'est pas?

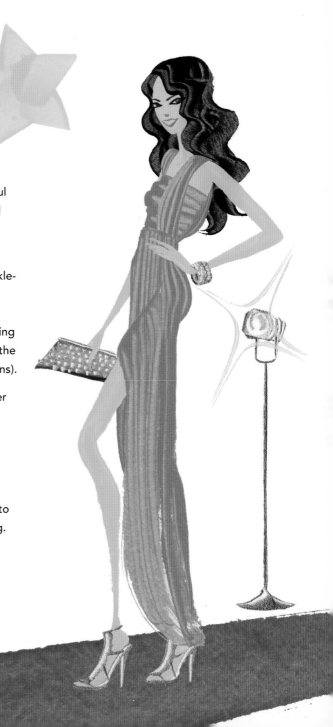

Run and splash

When you're lucky enough to spend a few hours at the beach or at a friend's pool, don't just lie around on your towel without moving for hours.

Stand up! Run on the sand, walk on the beach, jump in the water, play with the kids, play water polo in the pool, or even volleyball on the beach—a very intense activity, which can burn up to 500 calories in 1 hour. Lying around on your towel burns only 50!

LE PETIT SECRET *Grab a handful of damp sand at the water's edge and scrub your skin with it. Your skin will be soft as a baby's—and you'll have saved $100 at the spa! Bring some back home, mix it with almond or olive oil, and make a moisturizing scrub. (Make sure you rinse out the shower afterward so that the next person doesn't slip!)*

Move old magazines

Are you collecting tons of magazines about nutrition, fitness, and health? Put them to work! Relocate them on a permanent basis from one side of the house to the other— or even to the recycling bin. If you carry 10 magazines each time, using the biceps power in your upper arms and walking fast from one spot to the other, you'll shape your arms and burn quite a few calories as well.

QUICK TRICK!

Make sure you bend your knees when you lift those heavy magazines. You'll not only protect your back but will also build strong thighs.

"I never recycle magazines. They're a fitness tool!" —VALÉRIE

Supermarket trot

If you shop at a supermarket for groceries, you can ramp up your calorie burn by how you push the cart. Just push it as fast as you can and pull on the cart with your arms when you want to stop. As your cart gets heavier, you'll burn even more calories. So make sure you get the big bottles and cans first to add a few more pounds to your supermarket trot.

"Keep in mind that there's no speed limit in a store! Just watch those end-of-aisle turns!" —VALÉRIE

GRAB & GO! *Put the natural sweetener Stevia on your shopping list. It has no calories and tastes like a dream. Ditch the artificial stuff.*

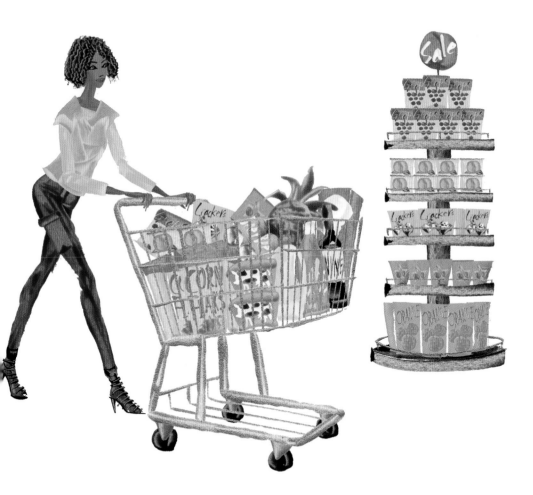

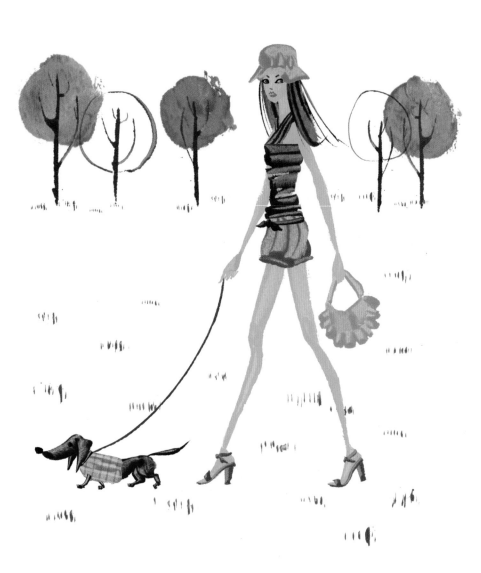

A bark in the park

A girl's best friend needs to go out several times every day.
And no one wants to breathe in all those exhaust fumes by
walking on sidewalks along a road. So pamper your fluffy friend
and go to a park. Once you snap on the leash, start with a slow
walk for a few minutes, then slowly accelerate the pace. Once
you're warmed up, how about a little trot? The idea is to get moving
together, because even your best friend needs to be in shape!

LE PETIT SECRET *Use the natural park
topography to vary your routine. Jump over a
rock, run along a river, run after a butterfly—if
you don't know what to do, let your dog lead!*

*"Many breeds, particularly small ones
with short noses, are susceptible to heat
stroke and exhaustion. Never ask any dog
to run when it's hot outside—particularly
on sidewalks or roads."* —VALÉRIE

Link to your bike!

Put your laptop or Blackberry on a stationary bike, then pedal for miles as you check Facebook, Twitter, or other social networks. You can get an extra hour of cardio each day—and burn 4 gazillion fat cells off your hips. If your electronics won't stay in place, check with your local bike shop. There are a slew of devices being made that will hold them in place as you pedal.

. . . .

Drop that jump rope!

Just leave it lying around your living room or in the backyard. Whenever you walk by, pick it up and skip rope 100 times. Fat cells will fall from your hips!

Find the stairs

If you're waiting for a doctor who's clearly scheduled far too many patients at one time, ask the receptionist to point you to the nearest flight of stairs. Then run up and down the stairs until your doctor's ready to see you. Not only will you condition your cardio system and burn calories, you'll burn off your annoyance at being kept waiting!

. . . .

Watch TV with your kids

Mais oui! But sit on a huge Swiss ball and bounce nonstop as you do. Not only will you have your delighted kids bouncing around you, you'll tighten your core and do amazing things for your thighs!

Park and hike

Whenever you take your car, park as far away from your destination as possible. Going to the supermarket? Park as far from the door as you can get!

GRAB & GO! *Remember how I told you to keep turkey jerky close at hand or in your car? Well, once you pull into a supermarket parking lot, get it out and eat it. Shopping hungry doubles what you'll spend!*

....

Get the drinks

Next time you go to a stadium for a baseball or football game, get tickets as far up in your section as you can. Then you'll have to climb up and down stairs and walk a few hundred feet to the refreshment stand!

Burn, baby, burn!

Toss an exercise mat on the floor beside your bed after your shower. Sit down with your weight on your tailbone. Then lift your legs straight out at a 45-degree angle, holding your chest straight (remember, no arching!) and your arms extended at eye level. Your body should be in the shape of a V, and your abs will burn from holding this position. Count to 30, then repeat twice in a row. Pretty intense, isn't it?

LE PETIT SECRET *Okay, you've just gotta have an Oreo. So go ahead. Eat one. Or two. Or . . . just pay the price. You can reverse the effects of 8 Oreos with 45 minutes of vigorous swimming, 30 minutes of spinning, 45 minutes of rowing, or 90 minutes on the treadmill at a normal walking speed.*

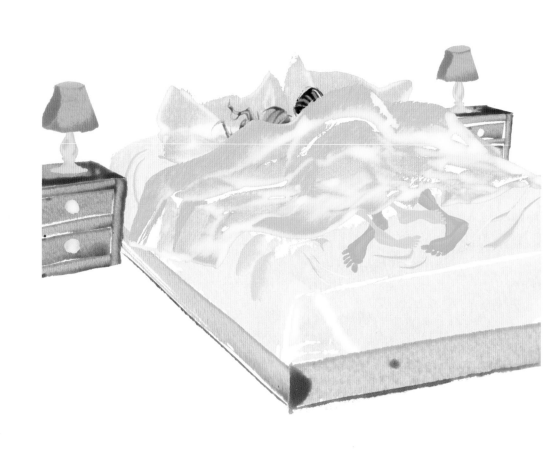

Work out in bed!

Hugging and kissing don't burn many calories, but a full-blown head-to-toe active and not-so-quick sexual encounter can burn up to 400 calories in an hour. Not as much as beach volleyball, but hey, who actually cares?

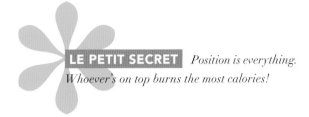

LE PETIT SECRET *Position is everything. Whoever's on top burns the most calories!*

Drive past the valet

Valet parking is everywhere. Initially only available at fancy restaurants, it quickly spread to chic shopping malls, resorts—and worse—gyms! Can you imagine? You're going for an hour of fitness training, and you can't even park your own car and walk 150 yards to the entrance?

I say NO! Next time you see a valet, don't stop and give him the car. Instead, park the car as far from the entrance as you can and walk.

"The only time to use valet parking would be if you were wearing very high heels. Walking 200 yards in a pair of those could kill your back!" —VALÉRIE

ST★R Rx

ADRIANA LIMA'S SLIM ANKLES

Having a toned body is nice, but who wants bloated ankles? Not Victoria's Secret model Adriana Lima. And not me, for sure!

One of the best ways to get fine ankles like Adriana's is to rotate them to the right and to the left at least 25 times every morning while still in bed, legs straight up, and before going to sleep at night. This will help get the fluid off your ankles.

A visual trick consists of toning your calves more so that your ankles appear smaller. Before climbing a flight of stairs, stand on the first step with your heels hanging over the edge. Shift your weight so that you stand on your tiptoes, hold it for a few seconds, then allow your heels to come down a little bit lower than the height of the stair. Do a quick set of 20 before climbing a flight of stairs—and again at the top.

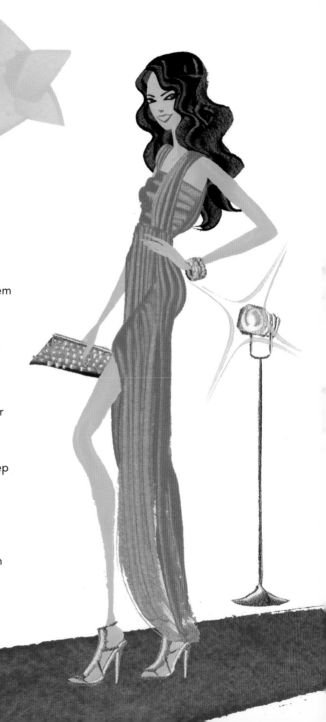

Inhale, exhale

If you've had a hectic day, chances are that you won't breathe properly. This leads to your being tired earlier than you should, which in turn leads to "No, I can't exercise today; I'm too tired."

Let's tackle the problem head-on. Every 30 minutes or so, take a deep breath, hold it in for 5 seconds, and as you exhale, slowly let go of all your toxic thoughts. Inhale again, visualize good things flowing in with your breath, hold it for 5 seconds, and once again, exhale all the bad stuff. Repeat 5 times.

LE PETIT SECRET *You'll create fewer wrinkles when you laugh than when you frown or sulk. It's a scientific fact!*

Ditch the restaurant line!

The next time you have to wait 30 minutes for a restaurant table, take a walk instead of having a drink at the bar. The walk will burn off a few calories before you eat—and you won't gulp down any extra ones from a martini or a soda.

"If I'm the first one to arrive at a restaurant where I'm meeting friends, I go outside and pace back and forth until they come. It's a great way to burn calories and zip up my energy for the evening!" —VALÉRIE

Weight that stroller

Pile bottles and heavy objects on the shelf underneath the stroller—and go for a walk. Adding weight to any physical activity greatly increases the number of calories expended. By adding weight to your walking, and power walking instead of ambling along, you can burn up to 600 calories an hour.

GRAB & GO! *Keep 5 almonds or other nuts in a snack-size plastic bag inside your handbag. Almonds send a strong signal of fat/protein intake to your brain, so if you munch on them before surrendering yourself to a slice of cake, your body will be less inclined to store it as fat.*

DO IT NOW! *Pile heavy stuff under your stroller when you walk and you'll lose every ounce you gained during pregnancy! If you power walk with your baby in the stroller once a day for 45 minutes, you'll spend the equivalent of 55 pounds of fat in a year!*

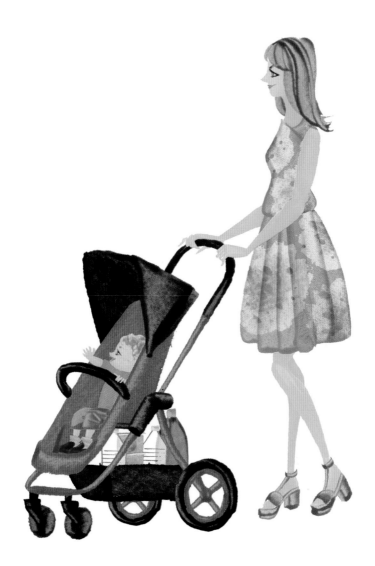

Work the magic triangle

Get killer inner thighs without leaving your comfy bed! Simply lie down on your back, arms along your body. Then spread your legs apart and bring them back together in one rapid motion, pointing your toes. Revert to the spread-out position and bring your legs back to center position.

When you perform the inward contractions necessary to do this move, make sure to put all your strength into them!

"Getting a model's thighs without getting out of bed—now that's a dream come true!" —VALÉRIE

DO IT NOW! *Visualize yourself in a bathing suit on a white-sand beach and go for it!*

Utilize boring ads

There are 10 minutes of television ads for every 30 minutes of programming on average. So instead of sitting on the couch drooling over fast-food ads, roll onto the carpet and lie flat on your back. Crunch up straight for 50 crunches, lie back, and then bicycle for 50 revolutions. Make sure your back is flat (no arching here), and suck in your stomach until it feels "glued" to the spine.

QUICK TRICK!

Up the ante. To tone the backs of your arms, do push-ups during TV ads. When an ad comes on, hit the floor and do 10 push-ups, rest, and stretch your arms. Repeat 4 more times before your program resumes. If your wrists are weak (like mine), then do girl push-ups, with your knees on the floor. It will still get you some nice results!

"Buy a rug for the TV room so you have no excuses to avoid crunches!" —VALÉRIE

Jump!

Start the day off right. Do 50 jumping jacks in the morning before breakfast and pump up your energy! Two minutes of jumping jacks will do wonders for your bone density. Just make sure you wear sneakers or shoes designed to cushion the shock of hitting the floor so hard. And if you're really, really overweight, don't jump—it will trash your knees.

"Jumping jacks are a great way to work off tension during the day. If you come out of a business meeting steaming or if the kids are driving you nuts, just go into a room by yourself and start jumping. You'll feel better within 2 minutes!" —VALÉRIE

DO IT NOW! *Jumping jacks will curb your appetite because aerobic activity is a natural appetite suppressant.*

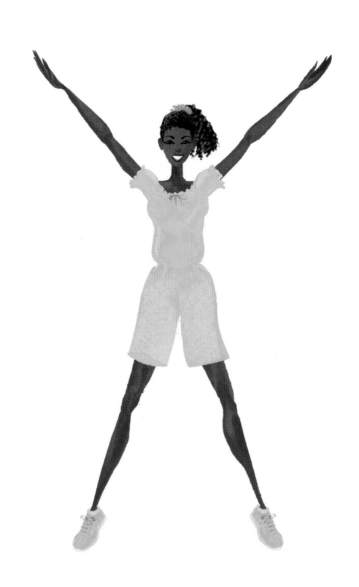

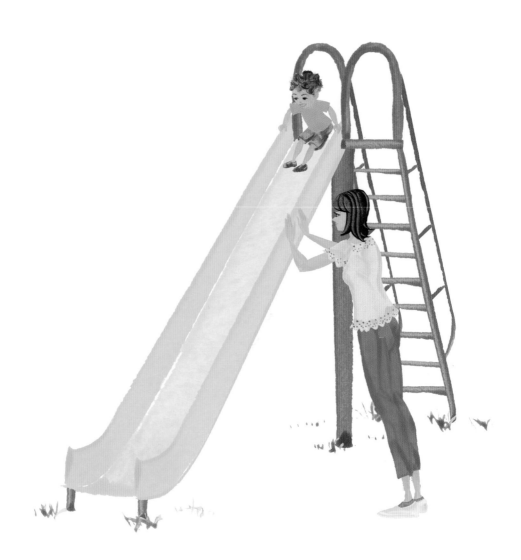

Head for the slide

Remember I suggested you take your younger kids to the playground? Well, as you wait for your child to come down the slide's slippery surface, do push-ups using the sides of the slide incline. Do as many push-ups as you can. Repeat until you've done 50. If you can't do 50 right away, start with 10 and gradually add 2 each day until you reach your goal. You'll be surprised how easy this is!

LE PETIT SECRET *Once your kids reach the bottom of the slide, go to the ladder, reach up, and grab the top rung. Use both hands and pull yourself up a few times as though you were doing a chin-up in the gym. It will really tone your arms—and your kids will want to see if they're as strong as Mommy!*

DO IT NOW! *If your children are overweight, why not make them part of your fun? They can do push-ups with Mommy before they get on the slide. And if they see you acting as a healthy parent, chances are, they'll try to become healthy, too!*

Reach for the sun

Put down a small mat beside your bed every night. When you wake in the morning, place your feet on the mat, face a sunny window, and gently raise both arms toward the sun. Stretch slowly upward until you're fully extended, then gently let your hands reach down to the floor and back up to the sun. Think of your hips as a hinge. Keep your legs straight when you reach up and when you reach down. And when you come back up after touching the floor, come up slowly, one vertebra at a time. Now you're ready in both mind and body to start your day.

"Before I start this movement, I open the window and draw in a deep breath of fresh air and focus my mind totally on my body." —VALÉRIE

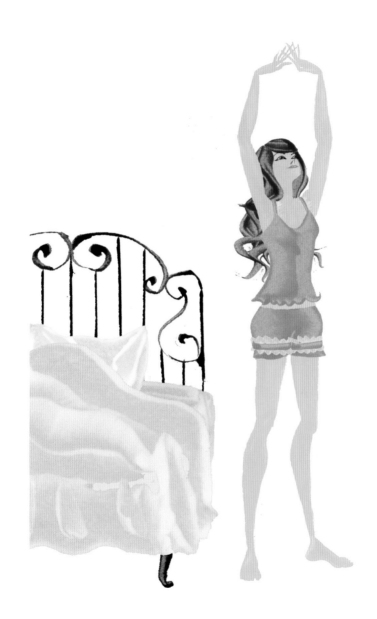

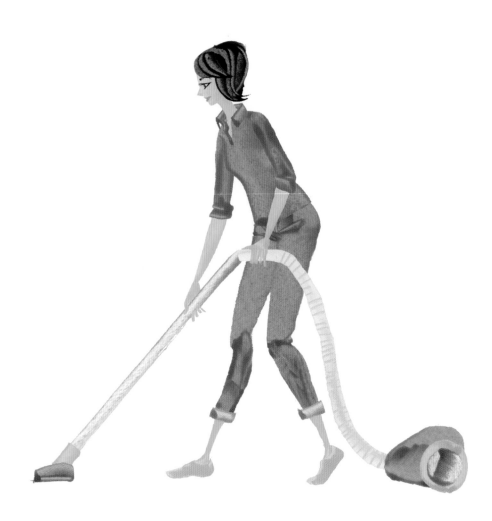

Fire the Roomba!

Robot vacuum cleaners are great, but vacuuming yourself at a fast pace for just 30 minutes will burn nearly 125 calories. So park the Roomba in its dock and pull the old upright out of the closet!

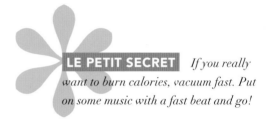

LE PETIT SECRET *If you really want to burn calories, vacuum fast. Put on some music with a fast beat and go!*

DO IT NOW! *If you vacuum twice a week for 30 minutes each time, you'll lose 1 pound of fat in as little as 14 weeks!*

Breathe!

If you wake up one morning facing a stressful day, start with some breathing exercises. They will not only help oxygenate your brain but also work on conditioning your diaphragm. The diaphragm is a critical element for efficient breathing. When we're stressed, we tend to breathe less deeply and therefore not use our diaphragm to its full capacity. This can generate a bloated feeling and stomach pain.

Inhale through your nose. Press your right thumb on your right nostril and exhale fully through the left nostril. Inhale through the left nostril. Remove your thumb from right nostril and put your pointer finger on your left nostril. Exhale deeply through your right nostril. Inhale and change sides to exhale. Try to do this exercise for 10 minutes.

The results will surprise you!

LE PETIT SECRET *You can boost lung capacity and liberate yourself from toxic emotions when you're driving in your car. Just play your favorite fast-beat song and sing at the top of your lungs. Keep the car windows up to avoid odd looks from fellow drivers!*

End interoffice e-mail

One day when I was working in corporate America, I decided to stop using e-mails to communicate with my colleagues down the hall. I walked instead. I walked 5,000 steps a day just by doing so—and I got to know my colleagues better!

"Visiting coworkers personally is one of the reasons <u>Outside</u> magazine named my company one of the best companies in America to work for!" —VALÉRIE

DO IT NOW! *Those 5,000 steps are a full half of the 10,000 steps doctors recommend you get every day to maintain a healthy body!*

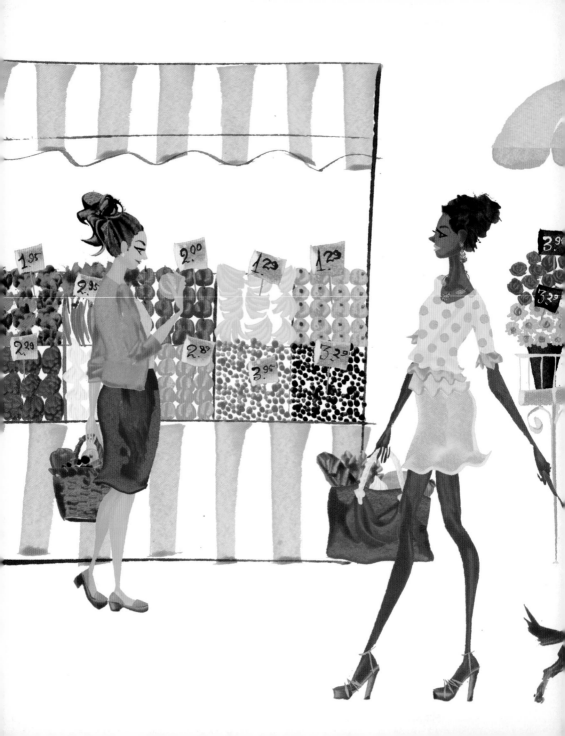

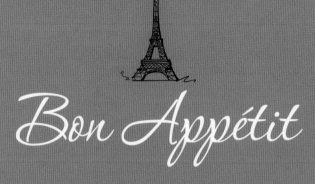

Bon Appétit

Oh-h-h-h! Grilled vegetables…a drizzle of rich olive oil…
a golden brown pastry…wild salmon…fresh strawberries…
coconut macaroons! I am a gourmand—a woman who
appreciates fine food, exquisitely prepared. But I can't
afford the calories of most restaurant offerings, and I
have no time in which to prepare exquisite food myself!
That's why I've developed a repertoire of quick recipes
that take minutes to prepare, give me the nutrients my
body needs to stay healthy, and provide me with sumptuous
foods that satisfy my passion for good eating. And although
I might not be willing to share a bite of my kiwi candy with
you, I am willing to share the recipe—and the recipes
for all my favorite high-energy, low-calorie foods!
Enjoy!

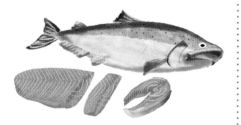
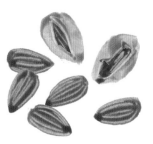
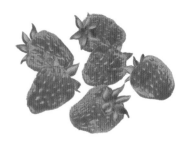
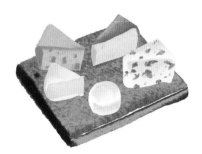
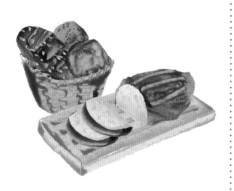
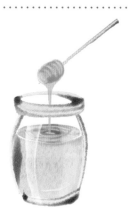

GREEN MORNING BOOST

*T*he *GREEN MORNING BOOST*, composed of spinach, celery, strawberries, and carrots, provides a powerful hit of the antioxidant quercetin and ellagic acid, which scientists suspect may slow tumor growth and help the liver remove cancer-causing subtances from your body.

1 apple

1 collard leaf or a handful of spinach leaves

1 celery stem

4 strawberries

1 carrot

1 fresh ginger slice

Rinse and pat dry all fruits and veggies.

No need to peel (except ginger root); you can put your fruits and veggies directly in the juicer.

Juice and drink right away, because antioxidants lose their potency as time passes.

SERVES 1

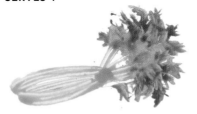

CREAMY STRAWBERRY SMOOTHIE

A smoothie a day may well keep the doctor at bay—at least if it's this strawberry smoothie! That's because tucked within the seductive taste of fresh strawberries is ellagic acid, a naturally occurring substance that scientists suspect may reduce your risk of cancer. Add that to the nice chunk of calcium found in yogurt, and you have a fabulously healthful drink!

1 pound (400 g) fresh strawberries

3 cups (510 g) natural yogurt

3 tbsp. sugar or no-calorie sweetener, such as Stevia

8 mint leaves, for garnish

Wash the strawberries and cut into pieces.

Place the strawberries, yogurt, and sweetener into a blender. Mix until smooth.

Pour into tall glasses and garnish with mint leaves.

Serve immediately!

SERVES 4

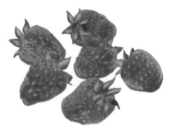

ALMOND MILK

Studies have found that a handful of nuts 5 days a week can cut your risk of a heart attack in half. They can also lower artery-clogging LDL cholesterol by 15 percent and boost the body's level of nitric oxide, a substance your body converts into something that dilates arteries and lets more blood reach the heart. You can always just eat nuts, but why should you when this almond milk is far more tasty? My son, who is a good test case, adores it!

1 handful of fresh almonds soaked in water overnight

1 tsp. vanilla extract (or less, if you prefer a less-distinct vanilla taste)

2 tbsp. agave nectar (from the agave cactus) or organic honey, available at specialty food stores or online

Banana or strawberries (optional)

The night before, soak the almonds in a bowl of water. Make sure the almonds are completely covered in water, because they will expand overnight.

In the morning, rinse and drain the almonds. Place in a blender, along with 2 to 3 times (or according to your taste) their volume of water.

Blend until the liquid turns white and milky.

Filter the milk through very fine filter paper or cheesecloth in order to eliminate pulp. Then discard the pulp. (I personally keep the pulp to make raw snack bars, but that's another story.)

To sweeten, add the agave nectar or honey. Drink immediately to benefit from all the vitamins!

You can also add some fruit—a banana or some strawberries—to make a tasty morning smoothie!

SERVES 1

HOMEMADE HUMMUS

This is a tasty and very healthy dip, side dish, or spread. I recommend you always keep it ready in your fridge to satisfy your salty/fiber cravings. My fave!

1 can garbanzo beans

½ lemon, squeezed

⅓ cup (79 ml) extra-virgin olive oil

½ tsp. tahini paste (sesame paste)

1 garlic clove

Salt to taste

Combine all ingredients in a mixer/blender and puree until smooth. Some people prefer it coarse. It is yours to choose!

To serve, put the mixture in a serving bowl. Pour some olive oil on top and garnish with a few olives, if you'd like.

VARIATIONS

- Add 2 tsp. cumin or paprika.
- Omit tahini paste (sesame paste).
- Add 1 cup fresh white mushrooms, finely chopped.

. . . Or be as creative as you want!

SERVES 4

GUACAMOLE

A *vocados are a great source of heart-healthy monounsaturated fats, and a recent study revealed that the fats in avocados actually contribute to the absorption of carotenoids—antioxidants found in bright red, orange, and yellow veggies. So having higher levels of these carotenoids in your body may actually help decrease your risk of heart disease and some cancers.*

Don't be shy! Enjoy your guacamole—but keep your portions under control.

2 ripe avocados

½ onion, thinly sliced

½ tomato (no seeds or juice)

10 cilantro leaves (also called coriander)

Juice of 1 lime

Slice the avocados in half, scoop flesh into a large bowl, and mash with a fork.

Add onion and tomato.

Cut cilantro leaves into thin strips and add to the mixture.

Add lime juice, mix once more, and chill until serving.

SERVING SUGGESTIONS
Eat with low-carb tortillas, as a spread in a sandwich, or as a condiment for grilled chicken.

SERVES 4

CELERY STICKS
WITH BLUE CHEESE

You can serve this dish with a slice of whole-wheat bread, grilled chicken, or baked ham (trimmed of fat).

7 ounces (190 g) celery stalks (cut into 3-inch/ 8-cm pieces)

1 cup plain yogurt

2.5 ounces (75 g) blue cheese

Salt and white pepper to taste

Slice the celery stalks finely and remove any strings if necessary.

In a pot, blanch the celery slices in 1 inch of salted water for about 2 to 3 minutes (no more or else they will lose their crunchiness). Drain and rinse under cold running water.

In a small bowl, mix the yogurt, blue cheese, and salt and pepper, until combined well.

SERVING SUGGESTIONS

The lazy approach: Serve the celery sticks in a tall cup alongside the cheese sauce.

The chic approach: Put 1 tbsp. sauce on each celery stick (like little boats) and place on a serving platter.

SERVES 1

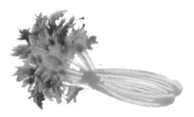

BANANA CHIPS

*O*ne of my healthiest tips for snacking and cravings, this recipe calls for a food dehydrator, but don't be concerned if you don't have one: See sidebar, "Simple Ways to Dry Your Food," on page 160 for some easy alternative drying methods.

2 bananas, peeled and thinly sliced

Lay the slices on a dehydrating tray.

Dry the banana for 12 hours at 100°F (38°C)—you could start your oven in the morning before leaving for the office.

Turn the slices and dehydrate for another 12 hours.

Remove from the oven. Let air dry before storing.

YIELDS 2 CUPS

TERIYAKI ALMONDS

*T*his is a great snack that you can eat on the go. Almonds are good for your health but also rich; hence, I recommend you eat only 10 per serving. Teriyaki sauce is originally from Japan. If you've eaten Japanese food before, you may have tried teriyaki eel or teriyaki chicken. Here's my version of a raw teriyaki recipe with soaked almonds loaded with beneficial enzymes. In this recipe I use Nama Shoyu, a raw soy sauce. You can find it in some organic and Asian stores or online.

2½ cups (375 g) almonds, soaked for 12 hours

⅓ cup (50 g) chopped dates (firmly packed)

¼ cup (120 ml) Nama Shoyu or soy sauce

1½ tsp. chopped garlic

1 tsp. finely minced fresh ginger

Rinse and drain almonds. In a food processor fitted with the S-blade, purée dates, Nama Shoyu, garlic, and ginger, until smooth. Toss the almonds in the paste and mix until coated.

Have ready one dehydrator tray fitted with both a grid and a nonstick dehydration sheet (see also sidebar, "Simple Ways to Dry Your Food," page 160). Place almond mixture onto the nonstick sheet and spread out into a single layer. Dehydrate at 145°F (65°C) for 1 hour. Turn the dehydrator down to 155°F (70°C) and continue dehydrating until the almonds form a skin, then flip them onto the grid sheet, peeling off the nonstick sheet. Continue to dehydrate until dry—about 48 hours total.

These teriyaki almonds keep well in an airtight container for about 2 weeks.

YIELDS 3 CUPS

Snack Cupboard

I don't believe in going hungry. So for those moments when my appetite says, "Let's eat," I keep the following on hand:

Few strips of turkey jerky or 98 percent fat-free beef jerky

1 cup low-fat cottage cheese sweetened with no-calorie sweetener, such as Stevia, or 1 tsp. honey

1 small piece mozzarella with 10 raw almonds

Homemade Chai Tea: Chai tea (tea bag) + skim milk + no-calorie sweetener or honey

1 slice whole-wheat bread with a small piece of Gruyere (a thin piece!)

2 slices honeydew melon

1 vegetarian burger with a slice of whole-grain bread

Broccoli or cauliflower with 1 tbsp. mayonnaise or, better, soyannaise

½ small packet peanut M&Ms (if you are in a movie theater and your craving gets the better of you). Opt for these because they have a lower impact on your glycemic index.

10 strawberries and 10 almonds

1 slice whole-grain bread with low-fat cream cheese

Celery sticks with a teaspoon of mayonnaise or, better, soyannaise

1 handful blueberries and 10 walnuts

½ of a cantaloupe with a small slice of prosciutto

1 cup (237 ml) whole-grain cereal + 1 cup skim milk

4 ounces (100 g) low-fat kettle potato chips

1 slice whole-grain bread with peanut butter or fresh almond butter (my favorite!)

1 green pepper cut into thin strips with hummus

1 soy yogurt

10 olives and ½ whole-wheat pita

1 apple

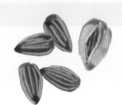

SALMON PIZZA

antalize your taste buds with this salmon dish. Salmon for omega 3, pita for fiber and B-group vitamins, tomato sauce for lycopene, etc.—a true benefit for you. Enjoy this dish in moderation, like all good things.

1 whole-grain pita

Pizza sauce

5 olives

1 ounce (30 g) reduced-fat mozzarella

Smoked salmon

A few oregano leaves

Pepper

1 tbsp. olive oil

Slice open the pita into 2 large circles. Place them with the inside faceup in an oven dish and heat for 8 minutes at 400°F (200°C), until slightly crusty.

Spread the pizza sauce over the inside of the pita slices.

Layer with olives, mozzarella, and smoked salmon.

Garnish with the oregano, a little pepper, and olive oil.

Place under the broiler in the oven until the mozzarella melts.

Enjoy!

SERVES 2

ZUCCHINI SOUP WITH BOURSIN

or a main course, you can serve this soup with 3.5 ounces (100 g) of shrimp, surimi (pollock), or smoked salmon.

2 zucchinis

4 ounces (113 g) Boursin cheese, or any other fresh herbed cheese (goat cheese will work well, too)

Salt and pepper, if desired

Rinse the zucchinis and cut in half. Place them in a pot with 2 cups of water and simmer, covered, for about 8 to 10 minutes until fork tender.

Pour the zucchini and its juice into a food processor and puree until smooth.

Add the cheese and pulse again until well combined. Season with salt and pepper, if desired.

Serve hot or cold.

SERVES 4

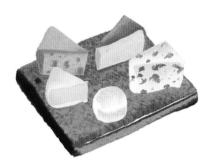

CARROT RAISIN SALAD

The vinaigrette in this salad is made with colza oil, which is known for its lovely fruity taste. Much lighter and more flavorful than oils that come from nuts and olives, colza is excellent in recipes that are uncooked, as well as in marinades and carpaccios.

4 large carrots

⅓ cup raisins

2 tbsp. soyonnaise

1 tbsp. balsamic vinegar

1 tbsp. colza oil

Parsley, for garnish

Grate carrots and put into a large salad bowl.

Add raisins and mix.

Prepare a vinaigrette with the soyonnaise, vinegar, and oil.

Add to salad and mix. Garnish with parsley.

Serve immediately before carrots become soft.

SERVES 4

GRILLED VEGETABLES EN CROUTE

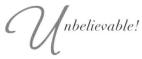 *nbelievable!*

1 puff pastry sheet

1 grilled eggplant, sliced

1 grilled zucchini, sliced

1 grilled red pepper, julienned

1 handful of spinach, cooked and drained

2 tbsp. olive oil

2 tbsp. black olive tapenade

Salt and pepper

Preheat oven to 350°F (175°C) for 10 minutes.

Generously butter a loaf pan. Line it with the puff pastry dough. Place one layer of each vegetable over the dough drizzling olive oil between the layers. Add the tapenade and season with salt and pepper. Repeat this until all ingredients are finished.

Wrap the pastry over the vegetables.

Transfer to the oven and bake for 20 minutes, or until the pastry is golden brown.

Remove from the oven and let cool before slicing.

Enjoy with a fresh green salad.

SERVES 6

FAUX MASHED POTATOES

*W*hat are faux mashed potatoes? They are mashed potatoes made without potato but with cauliflower and cheese instead. A true delight! Don't hesitate to make extra, because these mashed "potatoes" freeze very well.

1 cauliflower

2 tbsp. butter or Laughing Cow cheese

Salt and pepper to taste

Nutmeg (optional)

Steam the cauliflower until it can be easily mashed with a fork.

SERVES 4

While mashing, add butter or Laughing Cow cheese, salt, pepper, and nutmeg.

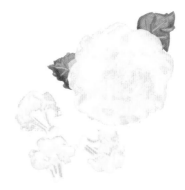

SMOKED SALMON ROLLS

T his recipe is perfect as an appetizer or first course. The salmon is rich in protein and good fat. I like to serve these rolls with fresh berries, which are an excellent source of antioxidants.

6 ounces (154 g) fat-free cream cheese

1 tsp. minced chives

Salt and pepper

Garlic powder (optional)

8 slices smoked salmon

In a small bowl, mix the cream cheese, chives, and salt and pepper. Add garlic powder.

On a plate, lay a slice of smoked salmon. Carefully spoon the cream-cheese mixture onto the salmon. Then roll the slice as you would for a spring roll. Repeat for the remaining slices.

Refrigerate until ready to eat. If served as an appetizer, slice up each roll into wheels and serve.

YIELDS 8

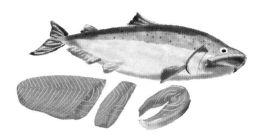

SEAFOOD RISOTTO

Like a day at the beach!

3 tbsp. olive oil

1¼ pounds (640 g) uncooked peeled shrimp

1¼ pounds calamari rings

1½ cups cooked rice

¾ cup dry white wine

1 cup (237 ml) chicken broth

Salt and pepper to taste

Pinch of saffron

Heat the olive oil in a sauté pan. Add the shrimp and sear them until nicely colored. Then set aside.

In the same sauté pan, briefly sear the calamari rings without cooking them completely.

Add the shrimp and cooked rice and simmer gently for about 10 minutes.

Add the white wine and chicken broth. Season with salt and pepper. Simmer until liquid is absorbed, stirring often.

The calamari and shrimp should be fork-tender.

Season with a pinch of saffron to give your risotto a nice color.

SERVES 4

WILD SOLE

Extremely simple to prepare, super healthy, and packed full of flavor.

3 sole fillets, preferably Dover or wild-caught

3 thin slices prosciutto

1 tsp. olive oil

Pepper

Juice of 1 lemon

2 tbsp. balsamic vinegar

Roll the sole fillets. Fold the prosciutto around each fillet to form a "belt."

Secure each fillet with 2 toothpicks and place in a roasting pan.

Rub with some olive oil and season with pepper.

Bake for 20 minutes at 350°F (177°C).

When the fillets are fully cooked, deglaze the sole juice with the lemon juice, balsamic vinegar, and a splash of water.

Place the fillets on a serving plate and drizzle with the sauce. Yum!

SERVES 3

WILD SALMON EN PAPILLOTE

One of my favorite recipes because of the omega 3's, this tastes great, is easy to prepare in its little parchment pouch, and is simple yet elegant. What more could you ask for?

1 salmon fillet, preferably wild-caught

1 tbsp. artichoke dip

1 tsp. whole-grain mustard

2 lemon slices

2 cherry tomatoes, halved

1 tsp. olive oil

Salt and pepper to taste

Parchment paper

Rub the salmon fillet with artichoke dip and whole-grain mustard.

Arrange the lemon slices and cherry tomatoes on top.

Sprinkle with olive oil and season with salt and pepper. Lay the fillet in the center of the parchment sheet. Fold it like a pouch and place the pouch on a baking sheet.

Cook in the oven at 350°F (177°C) for 20 to 30 minutes, depending on the thickness of the fillet.

SERVES 1

HERB-ENCRUSTED HADDOCK

The best! In this recipe I use almond flour (available at specialty food stores or online), which has the same great taste as pure almond extract, but without the alcohol.

3½ ounces (100 g) almond flour

1 tsp. curry powder

2 tbsp. chopped cilantro

2 tbsp. chopped parsley

Salt and pepper to taste

1 egg

4 haddock fillets, rinsed and dried

3 tbsp. olive oil

¾ cup (180 ml) whipping cream

Juice of 1 lemon

In a small bowl, combine the almond flour, curry powder, cilantro, parsley, and salt and pepper.

In a shallow plate, whisk the egg. Toss the haddock fillets in the egg and then roll them in the herb mixture.

Heat the olive oil in a skillet and sear each fillet, 4 minutes per side. Set aside and cover with foil.

In the same skillet, pour the whipping cream and let it reduce for 2 minutes. Add the lemon juice.

Uncover the fillets and place on a serving dish. Drizzle with the lemon sauce.

SERVES 4

COCONUT MACAROONS

*H*ere's a non-traditional spin on these delicious, sinful bites of coconut and maple syrup. I prefer to replace the maple syrup with agave nectar, available at specialty food stores or online. You will need a food dehydrator to make these macaroons.

Warning: *No more than 4 bites at a time! Can I trust you?*

3 cups (700 g) unsweetened ground coconut

1½ cups (350 g) almond flour (available at specialty food stores or online)

1 cup (200 g) agave nectar or maple syrup

½ cup (130 g) coconut butter or coconut oil

1 tsp. vanilla extract

½ tsp. sea salt

In a large bowl, combine all the ingredients and mix well. You can also use a standing mixer with the paddle attached.

Using a small ice-cream scoop, your hands, or a big tablespoon, spoon rounds of the dough onto dehydrator trays. If you are using your hands, it helps to refrigerate the mix for a short while prior to forming the macaroons.

Dehydrate at 155°F for 12 to 24 hours (70°C), or until crisp on the outside and nice and chewy on the inside.

SERVES 24

MOIST GRAPEFRUIT CAKE

rapefruit is an interesting source of antioxidants, protecting against many degenerative diseases and prolonging youthful skin.

1 yellow grapefruit, preferably organic

1 stick (125 g) butter, softened

¾ cup (150 g) confectioner's sugar

2 eggs

½ cup (115 g) flour

1 tsp. (5 g) baking powder

1 pink grapefruit, preferably organic

2 tbsp. Cointreau or any orange brandy

Juice the yellow grapefruit and place the liquid in a pot.

In a separate pot, blanch the zest of the grapefruit. When completely blanched, grate the zest.

Preheat oven to 180°C (350°F).

In a large mixing bowl, cream the softened butter with ½ cup (100 g) confectioner's sugar.

Add the eggs, flour, baking powder, grapefruit juice, and zest. Beat until fluffy and smooth.

Butter an 8-inch (20-cm) baking dish. Pour in the batter and bake for 35 minutes.

Let cake cool. Loosen the sides and invert into a deep dish.

Juice the pink grapefruit and combine its juice with the remaining confectioner's sugar and orange brandy.

Pour this mixture over the cake.

Once it's absorbed, garnish with some grapefruit pulp and serve.

SERVES 6

Simple Ways to Dry Your Food

If you don't have a food dehydrator, there are a few easy alternative drying methods. Whether you choose to dry your fruits, nuts, or vegetables outdoors, in a conventional oven, or on a solar dryer, you'll find the results will be delicious—and worth the effort.

Outdoors A hot, breezy climate with a minimum daytime temperature of 85°F (30°C) is perfect for drying sliced fruit in the sun. But if the temperature is too low or the humidity too high, the food may spoil before it is fully dried. Don't dry meats or vegetables outdoors because they spoil easily. You can fashion your own drying trays with food-safe nylon screening covered with cheesecloth to protect the fruit from birds and insects; place the trays on blocks to allow for good air movement. Be sure to flip the fruit regularly.

Conventional Ovens Your kitchen oven may take twice as long as a food dehydrator, and it isn't particularly energy efficient. However, you won't need any additional equipment, and it can be done in any climate. To start, set your oven to 140°F (60°C) and use cake-cooling racks placed on top of cookie sheets. Keep the rack with the trays 2 to 3 inches (5 to 7.5 cm) apart for air circulation.

Solar Dryers These dryers yield the same great results as dehydrators—without the electricity. However, they do require sunshine and high temperatures, and you'll need to assemble or build your own dryer. Many kits are available online.

KIWI CANDY

A little pleasure without the guilt, packed with vitamin C—now isn't that beautiful? This recipe calls for a dehydrator; for alternative drying methods see "Simple Ways to Dry Your Food," on the opposite page.

5 kiwis

Peel kiwis and cut each into 4 cubes.

Spread the slices on a dehydrator tray.

Keep in dehydrator for 6 to 8 hours at 110°F (40°C).

Refrigerate for a week and enjoy as a snack.

SERVES 5

Acknowledgments

One of my favorite pages in a book is the "thank you" page! I love to see who helped the author put it together. Who had to suffer endless sleepless nights, mood swings (yes, they do happen), and other predicaments that happen when one is fighting writer's block!

My first big thanks go to Reader's Digest France CEO Emmanuel Lecoq, for always believing in me and pushing me to publish in the United States. Thanks to his relentless energy and work, here we are! I must also disclose that Emmanuel knows how to feed me with freshly baked croissants when we need to talk about serious matters.

To my publisher, Readers Digest USA, I am indebted for life. Harold Clarke, you are my champion and the reason this book got published. You also gave me amazing Dolores York, who in her own words, took a whole village to make this book happen. George McKeon, Jennifer Tokarski, and Barbara Booth, thank you for making the words and images sing on every page. Rosanne McManus, Stacey Ashton—your creativity and availability are to be praised. And Ellen Michaud, you are amazing at understanding what a few scribbles mean!

To my family (Alex, Baptiste, Mom, and Dad), thank you for trying out my new exercises and toning/slimming techniques without complaining even when the postures were weird, to say the least. Your presence when I needed you most and your blind faith in me allowed this book to happen. Keep on believing in me even when I don't. It does make a huge difference between what can be done and what gets done.

To my amazing team at LeBootCamp & MyPrivateCoach, thank you for being creative whenever I asked the impossible from you, sometimes at crazy times. Anissa, you are irreplaceable. Sara, you rock and you are my rock. Toda raba. Gwen, Nadege, Marion, Marjorie, Edwige, you are truly one of a kind, and I want you to know it. To the geeks who surround me, thank you for having learned how to handle priorities when I ask for a new #1 priority right way: Eric, I know I get on your nerves sometimes with my 33k approach, but you seem to be holding on; Alex, you are the king of the Cloud, and you write the best code ever; Nicolas, you are so good at creating new designs; Denis, you proved that

Corsica exports not only good ham but also good engineers; Erik, you are good at saving me at 2:00 A.M. when things are truly urgent. I cannot cite all of you here, but you are in my heart.

To my bootcampers, famous or not, you are a wonderful source of techniques, since you always challenge me to find the routine that will do it. This book is dedicated to you!

To registered dietitians Gwenaelle Beau, Marion Bodin, Marjorie Faure, and Nadege Bedos in France. Thanks also to nutritionists Nathalie Hutter in France and Marge Mercury in Canada; physiologist Yomaho Yamamoto in Japan; nutritionist Denise Holz in the United States; fitness trainer Steve Barriere in both the United States and France; nutrition consultant Christiana Gopal in both Canada and India; certified herbalist Rivka Hecht in Australia; and last but not least, to Chef Ed, our in-house chef in France.

To the journalists around the world, who are reporting about LeBootCamp and its approach, you force me to become articulate each time I am interviewed, asking tricky questions, pushing me beyond my cocoon, and making me stretch my emotional fabric. Thanks to you I have learned a lot.

Thank you to Perez Hilton for being so prolific and entertaining. You have been part of my trips across the United States from one airport lounge to the other, where I read you on my PDA.

To Michelle Obama, your commitment to ending childhood obesity with so much energy and with so many efficient strategies and initiatives is an example First Ladies around the globe should follow instead of following the latest fashion trends.

To my publicists and agents—Leslie, Steve, Brooke, Gillian, and Danielle— you are taking good care of me. Love, always.

To Muse for its inspirational "Supermassive Black hole," Dan Black for "Alone," and Diana Gabaldon, whose *Outlander* series kept me awake when I needed to "blink blink."

And finally, to my friends with whom I work and play. You are here. You believe in me. I believe in you. We form an indestructible rock of friendship: Aline, Maud, Pascale, Selina, Tracey, Demi, Florence, Veronika, Sandrine, Nathalie, Paula, Mano, Clotilde, Véronique, Valérie, Britney, Isabelle, Marion, Kim, and the others. You are sometimes far away in miles but always close in my heart.

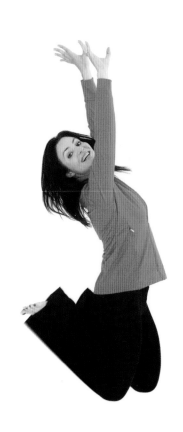